Rise of the Spiteful Mutants

The Death of the USA and Europe from dysgenics, feminism, and immigration

by

Pat R. Iotmouse

First Edition

Copyright (c) 2020 Makyo Press
All Rights Reserved
ISBN: 978-1-71692-207-7

Table of Contents

Introduction: Mutants Among Us..5
What is a Spiteful Mutant?...7
How Feminism Leads To Importing and Caring for Invaders........................13
The Cost of Dysgenic People and Spiteful Mutants.....................................19
When the Unintelligent Reproduce More than the Producers, What Fate Awaits the USA..25
The Life-cycle of the Feminist Woman..30
The Ice Age and Not Reproducing in Scarcity – It's In Our Genes..................34
Educating the Spiteful Mutant Children – Fake Degrees Fake College Fake Jobs, Taxes for the Producers...37
Genome Exhaustion After Being Conquered: Why Some Races Seem Terrible 49
Where are the Egyptians? Total Dysgenic Displacement of a Nation is the future the USA and Europe Faces...54
Modern "Egyptians" are a different people than the pyramid builders............56
The Dysgenic Effect of Divorce Rape..58
Life on the Tax Iceberg… Soon it will tip over..60
The New Baby Crisis...65
The Colluders – Plutocrats, MegaMillionaires, and the FED. Why you are going to be slammed and most big corporations are f-ed..............................73
Destroying the Intelligent Class: The H-1B Genocide Visa..................76
The Great Trump Failure and "Undocumented Neighbors".............................79
After the Red Pill Rage – Your Relation with Bythus – A Deeper Obscured Sacred that Wittgenstein told us about and Nan Chu'an Did Not....................81
The Debt, Higher Taxes, Inflation, Poorer Middle Class, Fewer Children Cycle 88
Absolutist Right – Dysgenics vs. Welfare, and Race — Which is the underlying principle affecting society?..91
The Extinction Party – The New Democrats and the End of America............96
Rise of the Dark State...99
How Welfare and Parasitism from Blacks and Invaders Impoverishes the Middle Class via Exorbitant Property Taxes..103
Psychopathology and Race..106
The Loss of the Europanic Peoples – No Homeland, Nowhere to Escape To, and the COST of the Spiteful Mutants will destroy us..................................113
Getting Europanic Women to have Babies in a Broken World 123
How to Face the Collapse of the USA ? 129
Conclusion: Two Futures Await Us..135

Introduction: Mutants Among Us

What are spiteful mutants? They are literally the population awash in negative genetic mutation, the lower herd, the adult babies on disability, the men wearing pink skinny jeans, and all of them whining and whining and complaining endlessly that they need moe more MORE free stuff because they do not produce or contribute.

They are childless barren women – we used to call them spinsters – who cackle and vision controlling others through thousands of namby complaints while wresting soul-lessly in mindless corporatia. Fed a diet of "you can do it" and feminism, they have rejected marriage and turned to whoring themselves for the first 30 years of their life, their egos haplessly fed by millions of single divorce raped men desperate not to be alone.

They are the affirmative action class heroes who live a comfortable middle class lifestyle in jobs they can neither do nor do they deserve.

They are the gender studies and african culture and basket weaving professors at Universities who earn six figures and leave your child's brain awash in mush and fake theories.

They are the invaders who sneak into America in the middle of the night anxious for their 20,000 dollar earned income tax credit and free housing, food and education. Even free breakfasts and dinners off the school lunch program while property taxes for American workers rise through the ceiling to pay for it all.

They are spiteful because they can never be happy. They are spiteful of the wealthy and hard working producer class. They prefer communism but not Russian communism, they like American communism where they get to sit on their duffs drink starbucks and eat chee-toes every day.

and sadly… they are US, they are what remains of nations like war torn Germany that lost its best and brightest and strongest men to war, or the US which simply has had its population replaced by immigrants seeking the welfare lifestyle. Or the non-Europanics who get pregnant endlessly as theres little else to do on welfare except thuggin and drug dealin. Being on the dole means you can't take a normal job. You'd lose your free housing and health insurance.

In short it is a madness we have created for our own nations through our own stupid government policies, and now after 60 years it's grown and bloated until they became us, they are our nation, they exceeded 50% of births, and it's only getting worse.

What happens when the productive class is only 20% of the nation? How does social security get funded? Who builds the roads, harvests the corn, and keeps the factories running. How do low IQ mental midgets become entrepreneurs with the creative force to fuel a nation?

This is their time to rise. And we are in the midst of them.

What is a Spiteful Mutant?

It's a complex formula that seems to include an abhorrence for real work, abusing the welfare system, and just plain genetic crap flowing through their veins.

It's not as simple as racial stereotypes. Mexicans in Mexico tend to be hard working family oriented people. That's not the Mexican we get up here in gringo stupido land.

I've met many blacks from Africa who were hard working and even entrepreneurial.

A key ingredient seems to be welfare and other government handouts gone wrong.

For example, an illegal invader from Guatemala with 3 children? Well her children get recognized as "DACANS" and get in state tuition and in California will get free health care insurance, school lunches breakfasts and dinners even during summer vacation. But it's worse than that. Let's take this example deeper.

She also gets a "Earned Income Tax Credit" and can backfile for two years. That's almost 20,000 dollars. She wasn't HERE in the USA those 2 years but prove that?

Many will get free housing and monthly cash for children, especially any children who are born here are considered "citizens" by the deranged commies. They aren't. But no one says they aren't. But they wouldn't get that IF they had too much income from their husband. So their husband is never declared. They just illegally state they as. a single woman.

The husband works for cash in construction, mowin lawns, restaurant work, whatever they can find. The welfare gets them a base equivalent salary to a hard working American earning $60,000 a year. PLUS they get the husbands income.

This lax morality is racial. Smaller lesser developed brains often completely lack a moral compass. Many nations in Africa have such limited language they don't even have the words for a morality. The pakistani filing bogus medicaid claims for a business, or taking an elderly bus from a nursing home then billing for 20,000 in tests on each of them... wham bam moneygram.

The thing is, while it's true that Europanics also can be criminals, you just don't see this "lets scam and rape the country" except out of the banker/financial mba asshat class. Regular workin' folk would never dream of doing such things.

Take a group of 500 Germans 500 Italians and 500 Irish and put them on welfare. Check back in six months later and they will all be gone, finding productive lives. So why can't the other races do that? There are genetic components not just for IQ and Psychopathology, but most likely there are alleles for work ethic, determination, and striving. Sure, if you get taught by your father to be self reliant you might pick up on it early on, but I never had that and I refused death-fare over and over and made something of myself from the poorest urchin. So why can't blacks? So why not our Hispanic Invaders? Why does the Pakistani gather gangs to rape little girls? Welfare is a contributing factor to decline, but there is also the other side the susceptibility to accepting a life of sloth on the dole.

To be a spiteful mutant, you must also be spiteful. You hate the country that took you in. Sounds like a few of those congresswomen from muslim countries that faked being part of a family to get in. Listen to them, they spew hate. It's the Andrew Cuomo "America was never great" horror. Leftism, which is no more than communism and nutcases seeking total fascist control push this hating the nation which saved them endlessly. It's the rhetoric of the day on television.

You can be a spiteful mutant even if you are in the upper half of society. Bitter college students scowl that the world seems to ignore them and "the man" keeps em down. Its a whole psyche that's destroyed with broken ideas that only lead to failure but are pushed on our poor children since birth. A misunderstanding of equality (Jefferson meant Not KINGS not all men are equal). A watered down commie drivel. A victim-hood identity. Left handed aqualung wearing Amerinds who dislike hopscotch. It doesn't matter what it is, its a lie to set up a us vs. them society, and ultimately is drive by the upper level commies who want nothing more to bring down society so they can rule not as commies, but ABSOLUTELY (think STALIN then LENIN).

Even a native Europanic can be a spiteful mutant. The adult baby on disability in Seattle, the man in the pink skinny jeans at the coffee hut. They confuse normal borders and rational population growth with a Zieg Heil Nazism which even Hitler never performed. Don't get to close or they'll throw coffee or a concrete milkshake on you and call you a Nazi or a Hater, lefty code for Patriot.

But we know all this. We have spiteful mutants among us. And soon, a majority of them. We have been slow sinking in quicksand and some dumbasses think just because our head is still above and can breath that all's ok. It's not. We're about to go under, and plenty quick.

Spiteful mutants are spiteful because they lack cognitive ability. They are the lower herd, the mad masses. They are zombies. They have had their midget minds twisted. they think there's nothing wrong at all with ripping everything off cause "its all free in America" reminds me of the people who waited for "obama money" and to get their rent and student loans paid off. they are still waiting.

In terms of the races we know, some races seem to have much more psychopathology than others and lower IQ (see Richard Lynn's seminal works). That shouldn't shock you. When I was younger it was common thought that other races were backwards and needed help – we called it the white man's burden. Today that concept of being OUR burden has broken our nation, sent us into trillions in debt, and doomed our nation.

If you ARE a non-Europanic race, remember Europanics invented ALL of the modern world. All of it. The Chinee just stole the inventions. The Japanese just made them cheaper. But anything you can NAME was invented by Europanics. And some Jews. Who really, are mostly europanics with that Kazar legacy. Is it racist to say the truth? In this world today, it is. But that begs the question if the truth is racism, then what the heck is racism? But the point is, just because you are non-Europanic does not mean as an individual you are condemned. Even if you aren't blessed with a high IQ, work ethic, inventive ethic, and normal pathological rates. You can still do your best and succeed quite well. It's really the group means that are so abhorrent. wait, I can't say that it's racist. Unfortunately its very much the truth.

Calling someone WHITE is quite racist actually. People of Europanic origen, aka Europanics is preferred. But no one cares what we want people to call us. Once you say "white" you have adopted a racist tone. We don't call asians "yellows" and amerinds "reds" although we used to. Blacks are still black, but they aren't black any more. More like a pallow gray. I've seen some real blacks from Africa and they aren't what we have here. the Kamala Harris black worries me. The kapernic black worries me. These diminutive genetically blacks with perhaps 10% blackhood seem to riot against and hate Europanics in an effort to be included in black world. Why don't they struggle to be recognize as whites? Because all the gibs go to blacks not whites. Free college, affirmitive action, just ask Elizabeth Warren she got into Harvard and made millions just for lying and declaring herself amerind. Wish I had done that, but I could not, again, my MORAL COMPASS won't let me which is why Warren is such a hated shrew by Europanics. But she's loved by feminista women, which are the OTHER class of spiteful mutants.

The feminista women, often Europanic women, often CODDLED AND UTTERLY SPOILED through life, are often the most vile mutants of all. They have been sold a lie that will lead to their destruction as a cat Karen alone in her 40s. The government pays for their abortia and their bastard children. Or they divorce rape men. Leaving ever more men desperate to find a companion, which skews the dating pool causing women to think they are the great prizes. They aren't. Far from it they are a horror, a slave chain, willing to divorce rape a man and take 75% of his savings and earnings without a whit of care that he might off himself with a government proclamation that his life is to be destroyed for all time. What did he do? Well see, the woman got "bored" and chad and tyrone on welfare were just having fun all the time so the hard working career male just isnt as much fun anymore. Others think their 20 something chad-ster is actually in love with them. Often he's just another mooch on the chain. After the divorce rape he will be her steed while the divorced husband pays for their life together. And she will cackle and hate her ex husband with her every breath. It's another spiteful mutant case, except that shes feeding off a cucked husband. Our nation changed the laws. Handed everything over to women and set up kangaroo divorce courts to take everything from men. Don't get me started on METOO. Why aren't Europanics having children? You'd have to be pretty dumb to fall for this enslavement system. The best and brightest walk away, the betas still get a woman pregnant and end up getting his money siphoned off for the rest of his life until he breaks and dies.

So when, through immigration, communism/demothugs, welfarism, and feminism grows out of control, and the population of these spiteful mutants exceed 50% of the population, your nation is headed towards doom. Already the only reason Europanics are greater than 50% is because of our older people, the younguns are already named Muhammed or Chad or Jesus is big numbers. In the elementary schools already its 70% mutants. So that means its only 10-20 years before the whole nation dies. But until that happens they will feed on our largess and welfare and divorce rape and cause the government to run out of money. The government will print money out of thin air, and inflate away the value of our currency to nothing. Social security goes broke in 2035. Thats 15 years. That may be optimistic.

How Feminism Leads To Importing and Caring for Invaders

Feminism has been a driving force in a misplaced "care" morality. Child-less Spinsters feel a need to "mother" and adopt invading illegal alien adults and children of a different race and culture. Many try to specifically do so (see all the articles of Hollyweird nutcase female actors who bring on the black adoptions – Brad Pitts wife comes to mind)

This happens because their female instincts have always been to protect the tribe. during the ice ages, survival was critical. Women played a critical role in nurturing and caring for the children. These instincts were genetically encoded. Everything went great until…

Women LOST THE ABILITY TO RECOGNIZE THEIR TRIBE.

It's true. Being constantly surrounded by peoples of other tribes – blacks, asians, mehicanos, they somehow forgot they were Europanic peoples. But the urges to protect and nurture remained. Thus, without them even knowing it, they began to push for an insane agenda of helping other races to invade and take over, and caring for them when they did so.

Take the recent case of the female Seattle Mayor:

> Seattle leaders called on the Washington state government to establish a coronavirus relief fund that provides millions in cash assistance to illegal aliens.

> The Seattle City Council passed a resolution Monday encouraging Democratic Gov. Jay Inslee and state lawmakers to establish a Washington Worker Relief Fund to "provide emergency economic assistance to undocumented Washingtonians," according to the Seattle Times.

Woe to the poor invaders who RAPED our nation sneaking in and breaking our entrance laws breaking our identification laws, forging federal documents, and being uncontrollable because they live under assumed names many hiding from criminal pasts back home. Nope, we gotta help them, cause that's the feminist genetic.

> City councillors are calling attention to illegal aliens in the state who do not qualify for federal assistance because of their immigration status, but have been suffering due to the declining economic conditions brought on by the coronavirus pandemic. The measure suggests the Washington Worker Relief Fund should begin with an initial allocation of $100 million.

To them, the invaders rapists murdering thuggies are just "their tribe". The word they use is "community". They see themselves as protectors and encouragers, to care for them all.

With zero mental ability to grasp the concept that these are DESTRUCTIVE ANTI-TRIBE forces.

> "Looking out for the most vulnerable in our community is even more critical in times of crisis," Seattle Mayor Jenny Durkan said in a Monday statement.
>
> The measure sailed through the city council by a vote of 9-0, and enjoys support from the mayor's office.

Thus it begins. Herds of unmarried communist demothug women without children adopt the invading and social malcontents and push policies to feed clothe and shelter them. More welfare, more freebies, because they are our tribe of course. Taxes to pay for all of it impoverishing our true tribe? No problem! Because we are all one WORLD tribe.

Somehow my brain hasn't made that adjustment at all yet.

We are in a fight between feminist agenda false tribe recognition and ice-age laden genetics which will destroy any country that takes it up, and the freedom tribe recognizing people. When America was 90% Europanic it was obvious what tribe we were. But then the women got suffrage and soon EVERYBODY was our tribe. The chinee rail workers. The blacks. America was a "melting pot" except, genes don't melt. No, the Europanic gene is recessive when mated to other dysgenic races, it loses dominance and the brilliant inventive world creating dynamo that is the Europanic race fizzels out with all the mulatto babies.

This happened with the moor invasions of southern Italy. To this day the southerners are seen as more dim, coarse, and unproductive than the north, and their phenotype shows the non-europanic admixture. And that is only with slight mixing. We can look to India and Egypt to see what happens when the dysgenic blender takes effect. Entire nations missing their founding peoples. And now America is on that same path, apparently clueless or to social justice warrior to be able to speak the truth.

There is simply no way to change or educate the women on this point. Somehow it was never required evolutionarily to detect who was their tribe, their tribe simply was around them. Give it 10,000 years and they will develop the alleles for it, but by then of course we will have been destroyed 1000 times over.

So if the women are helpless, it's up to the MEN to step up and lead. Why isn't this happening? Because we live in a Gynocracy where women hold the chains of command and the few men in power kow-tow to them. Can you say IVANKA? It was Ivanka and simp Jared who changed Trump's idea to block immigrant visas during the covid crises. They made sure the H-1A and H-1B invaders got to keep coming, destroying job prospects for American engineers. Why? Because they have NO CONCEPT that they are being anything more than loving. Another issue with most women's smaller brains is they lack logic / deductive reasoning, certainly they are allowed to skate through an education system never developing it. So rarely do they have a sense of consequences. They have an emotive response. The demothugs capitalize on this and it's all emotive propaganda, and little if ever any logic or consequences. "We must spend 300 trillion or the climate will change" err.. climate has been changing since I was born sista, what are you harping about.

This is not to say ALL women. It's a bell curve with a tiny segment achieving high IQ/productive levels. It's as if there should be a test and if women can't pass it go back and make babies. We need the babies. We don't need emotive care based morality forcing higher taxes and American bankruptcy to pay for invaders, rapists, and thuggess from around the planet. Yes it may make you feel good. But it's killing people for Christsake!

Loss of a tribe is one way the government tries to control all of us. We don't have the same open gathering spaces, even open parks that there once used to be. The few spaces that exist – bars – have televisions blaring with sports (propaganda for a fake tribe for MEN to join).

For men the fake tribe is the sports team. And they have such longing to belong many fall for it. Get suckered into a game that means nothing rather than focusing on matters in the real world. These are the zombie beta cucks. The chest thumpers. The life wasters. It's all a time suck cheering for people who often aren't even in your tribe at all. Yet they get millions. Because mind control is very very important. Sports fulfills the competition allele that men are programmed with. Rather than compete in the real world. It fulfills their innate "defend the tribe" allele rather than defending their tribe in the real world. This is why things have progressed to such a state. Break the sports hypnosis and maybe they can wake up. But so many are so weak minded.

For women, tribe often becomes a church or charity group – helping. Which is what their allele to care tells them to do. It's all exactly as planned except, it's not their tribe. I went to a food bank once. Big brand new SUVs pulled up. "how many in your household" they asked the mexican man. "24" he replied. They carried half the food out of the place in their brand new SUVs.

When I finally got called "sorry we are out of meat" and I got one old stale box of mac and cheese and some crackers. This is what happens when women who have no sense of tribe run things.

The Cost of Dysgenic People and Spiteful Mutants

So Europanic population in America was 90% in 1960. There was a surplus going into the social security system and deficits were slow growing mainly caused by war spending.

We were able to support the 75% of negroid race that was dysgenic and the 20% of the white race that was dysgenic. About 20% of the whole population. The working 80% were more than enough to produce enough excess to provide for all of them who were non-productive net users of resource.

But fast forward to today. We have spent the social security excess and soon will have a cost of 200-400 billion a year to cover that. The hoardes of immigrants going on disability have bankrupted the disability fund and now are being paid out of the general social security fund. Bankrupting it.

We suffer a unbelievable dysgenic load. The Europanic load remains at 20%, but now with 45% dysgenic races in America – blacks amerind and hispanic, produce another 30% dysgenic population. So the total dysgenic load is now 50%. One productive person can only support at most one non-productive and at that level the support will be very low. Our current level of dysgenic horror is now running at 6.5 trillion in 2017 represents an exhausting tax rate. This leads to Europanics forsaking family formation and marriage and their reproductive rate is at an all time low far beyond replacement. This is due not so much to external factors, it is mostly the huge strain produced by heavy taxation and the unaffordibility of the middle class life.

We now have over a TRILLION dollars a year in debt. But to be honest, let's add the 500 billion that Europanics are paying into the social security system which get spent instantly. This is very telling. Even at 65% Europanic race the system cannot support the dysgenic races huge handout system.

If we look at the homocide rates in major cities (murder is the only statistic that all agencies are required to report) there is a clear correlation between dysgenic population and homocide rate. For example Baltimore, a modest sized city of 650,000, and which has several major universities such as Johns Hopkins, has a 28% Europanic vs. 67% Dysgenic race profile. It's homocide rate is off the charts at 44/100,000 per year, or 275 homocide deaths so far this year. Chicago, a very strong industrial American city, the third largest, has a 31.7 Europanic population and 60% dysgenic race. It's homocide rate is a whopping 29 per 100,000 (source Wikipedia) or 507 deaths three quarters into the 2017 year.

Atlanta, a very cosmopolitan city with large companies such as Coca Cola calling it home, has the huge homocide rate of 13 per 100,000. 111 murders in 2016. It has a Europanic population of 38% (2010 census) and a dysgenic racial population of 60%.

It's shocking to see that such major cities in America are majority non white. Austin Texas is one of the cities that has the lowest homicide rates in America, for a million person sized city. It has a 43% dysgenic population but of that only 8% is black. The city is 50% non-hispanic white. It's more strict social policies means that much of the Hispanic population are productive workers. It's murder rate per 100,000 is only 2.5.

Even if the load were decreased by half, we would never approach affordability. Now project the USA reaching 50% Europanic we can project a doubling of our deficit each year throwing our debt into the hyperbolic and most likely the utter fiscal collapse of the nation.

So we only have two paths. Either the US adopts a government policy which redirects our dysgenic race proportionality BACK to near the 1960s level (say 15% dysgenic, not 50%) or our nation will utterly collapse. Well you can't just exterminate everyone but that is what Liberals think is the only option when you start discussing dysgenics. There are actually several paths forward. Immigration controls both in blocking welfare to immigrants, not counting foreign births as citizens, a racial immigration quota system which hugely favors Europanics, promoting the breeding of the best of the dysgenic races not the worst (aka welfare queens with 8 children), promoting the breeding and offspring of our best Europanic citizens, and government dynamic response to ensure we are indeed reversing our dysgenic racial profile and making success every year and taking further measures.

The system which allows and rewards with free money and housing those who never strive to achieve fiscally or intellectually and simply impregnate themselves in high school so that by the time they are 16 they have three babies and require total support for the government while having paid in nothing has to be utterly overhauled. How much help you get back if you have a time of need should be based entirely on how much you put into the system. So if you never ever have worked, which is the scam many of these black teens aspire to, and think simply by having children out of wedlock you will be granted a free life equal to a hard working 60k a year professional, well that has to end and end now. If you have never paid in, you should receive only a meager pittance enough for minimal food. And no free housing period. The section 8 horror which allows our poor to live in identical housing as our hard working classes is ridiculous.

Perhaps we can build some concrete bunkers with 100sq foot living spaces for the poor.

"You're so mean and unfeeling" say the liberals. The liberals have defective brains incapable of teleological thinking and fiscal analysis. For them the whole world is free (probably they were raised that way!) and you can show them chart after chart which prove the cost of the dysgenic races and they will still go on talk shows and argue that immigrants are a net benefit. They will mention Sergey Brin who arrived at age 6 was Russin (white) and highly intelligent. This is NOT the profile of the dumb african and middle eastern horrors who flood our shores and have wreaked a devestation of violence and rape in Europe and are overwhelmingly still on government assistance. These are not the high IQ hard working immigrants from Italy France and Germany who came to America in the beginning of the 20th century.

To re-establish high IQ base citizens at a 75% of population will require additional measures most likely including breeding programs. Women of good intelligence and character should be able to choose to enter a breeding program where they produce and raise 10 children each in exchange for a guaranteed high level of government support for their entire lives. Men would be chosen from the elite universities and based on their program of study and achievement, as well as older males who have exceptional achievement. It might take 2 or even 5 million women to enter these programs, it would be vast. But we would simply redirect the monies from welfare handouts to dysgenic races, to supporting increasing the children of the pro-genic races. Older women who need retirement assistance can volunteer to be nannies and helpers as each larger family is raised, and the original fathers would be required to spend time teaching their children. It's not quite marriage, but it's better than single motherhood. As women insist on outrageous divorce settlements and the courts give it to them, we may have no choice but to consider such seeming odd for us measures. If you think about it, welfare queens with 8 children (or 20! see "somebody's gotta pay for all my children" article) we are doing it today but in the reverse direction.

The next question is who qualifies? Do Jews? Do half blacks? Do mixed race people who are 50% white 50% asian qualify? This is a tough question. The simpler answer of only allowing traditional Europanic races is a likely start.

The other question, as we slowly return to a highly productive intelligent nation, will we restrict some states to white only. The beautiful west coast states of California, Oregon, and Washington have been utterly destroyed by the dysgenics. It's time to return them. Watch movies of San Francisco shot in the 1950s and you will be amazed. It seems like an idyllic society beyond belief.

What about the Chinese and Indian restaurants? What about all that multi-culturual gravy? Well, in Portland, the best Thai resturant is run by a Europanic chef. Over in Europe Swedish chefs prepare American cuisine. We don't have to return to the banal culturally limited food or films or crafts. All of it will still be available. In fact only some of the dysgenic races seem to be any good at all at starting businesses. In all Europanic states we can produce just as much creativity.

If we are wrong about the dysgenic races then we ask, where is the example of a state run by them in the world that is a success? South Africa, Zimbabwe all fell to hell after Europanics departed. We don't want to bring that hell to America. The Genetic potential of every race is not the same, something the Left Liberals are incapable of realizing with their non-science brains.

All of the wasted money on closing "gaps" in achievement due to some false sense of egalitarianism are all utterly based on false pretenses. We never try to do the same with the NFL and NBA lineups. All of this misdirected energy and money could be redirected to finally helping our high – IQ youngsters who are often ignored.

The dysgenic challenge seems frightening, Hitlerian, impossible. But if we do not solve it, we will utterly be destroyed. So what choice do we have but to consider this as the way modern societies MUST EXIST. There may be separation there may need to be advanced fertility control devices implanted at age ten. And certainly it's hard to trust the state to run anything correctly. We need to change course in the very near future. So we need to start the difficult discussion now. Yes they will scream RACISS DAS RACISS. So be it. It is in fact RACIAL, but not racist. It is based on science, fact, and reality. It is not based on an irrational belief. The KNOWLEDGE that other races are dysgenic, the huge body of knowledge, study, and research is now utterly incontrovertible. So what would they have us do deny our intelligent analysis? This does not come from some HATE or PREJUDICE it comes out of actual understanding of the terrible consequences especially FISCAL LOAD which occurs when we are increasingly bound with larger populations of dysgenic races. WE can deny the path we are on and utterly die and decend into HELL (just look at DETROIT or COMPTON for an example) or we can take intelligent measured action. Debate it. And prosper. And this prospertity is for all peoples of all races – everyone will be lifted up. If not, everyone will descend to near starvation, cities full of rape and crime and terror. It is our path to chose, if you fall to political correctness you doom our entire race.

When the Unintelligent Reproduce More than the Producers, What Fate Awaits the USA

> During most of history intelligent people became more prosperous than unintelligent people, and had more children who survived and reproduced. Intelligent people still tend to become more prosperous than unintelligent people, but they no longer have more children. Welfare checks enable extremely unintelligent women to give birth to future welfare recipients.

This is what I call Dysgenics in a nutshell. It's reverse Darwin, where the least fit survive to reproduce.

Sadly it's the state of America for many decades now. We are going into reverse as a nation.

It's not simply whose having the kids, it's admitting MILLIONS of dysgenic peoples into our country each and every year. Low IQ Indians, Government Quisling Chinese, and make a good taco Mexicans. Wait I love Mexicans. They do GREAT in their own culture. In Mexico. They are well adapted to work and thrive there. But put them into welfare-stato USA and they become kids filling up our schools, grannies crowding emergency rooms, and budget draining welfare suckers. All the worse due to anchor babies – the fake citizens that no one seems to call out.

How did this happen. Moreover, why do we stand for it?

We do not wish to appear Goshe. That's it. That's the reason for our entire economic collapse as a nation. It's tough to be sanguine when one studies the situation clearly. We are hurling straight for the cliff like a freight train, all the charts show it.

It's a population flip, when the dysgenics overturn the productive contributers in size. We are seemingly weeks away from that happening, it's already happend in the birthing wards and schools. Does no one care or are they still trying to win brownie points for calling me a racist?

Moreover, what can be done. Do we do a Aaron Cleary sit back and enjoy the decline, try to laugh? We do need a new homeland. Sadly, we are the last one to fall there's no where else to go. Now that governments have machine guns and arial bombs, it's hardly likely I can take them on from my small tent.

Welfare can never be turned off but it can be MODIFIED. Reward them for NOT HAVING CHILDREN with a bonus check. If they sign up for tube tying they get more. Instead we pay them MORE for each child. Madness. We also give them priority to get free housing the more kids they have. You think the black 15 year old high school girls don't know that. Of course they do. they know they need to get up to 3 or 4 chillin before big moma throws em out if they want section 8. And on it goes. Well its the crappiest of Europanic people as well, blacks aren't the only ones on welfare they are simply the most egregious.

So why is the government so bad? Well because the billionaires are so bad. Why are they so bad? They feel guilty over getting so rich so they push a destroy America policy. That's nuts you say. IT IS I reply. and nothing changes.

So real change will happen when we form a THIRD political party and not before. Sure Trump spoke platitudes, then didn't prosecute Hillary (remember Lock Her Up?) didn't declcare anchor babies non citizens and didn't really do much except spend ridiculously on an already fat stuffed military and then gloat on it 5000 times.

Population movements away from the Democratic strongholds is already well underway. We simply have to block the invaders from taking our empty seats AND have a census that doesn't count illegal aliens – Another issue Trump caved on.

What about stopping Election fraud. Another issue trump caved on.

The Trump lesson for us, was even when the politico says ALL THE RIGHT THINGS they still betray us. There is no way to remain a demothug or a plutocrat after this.

And for the slightly older, retirement is impossible in America with no true property ownership – effective communism, where the property taxes make you feel UTTERLY UNSECURE your whole life. And that's precisely what they want. Why can't I buy free land in a town in this nation. Nowhere? I think some barren desert scrub in west texas where your nearest neighbor is 20 miles off and hes a billy goat is about all this nation has to offer. ICK!

Not for me, I'm headin' off to Mehico. I'd rather be with the productive beaners than the lazy ones.

SAT scores are dropping but don't seem dramatic yet, even after they rewrote the test to help dumber students. But you have to understand that the SAT is a filtered class of students. The dumb students don't take the test or have already been pushed out of High Schools for being too violent.

There is also rampant fraud with the test.

In the end, as long as our spiteful mutants continue to breed like rabbits on welfare, and slong across our borders legally and illegally to the tune of THREE MILLION a year (1%) yet have 70% of our babies, it's only 20 years from a IQPocalypse.

America continues to shit on its best and brightest, using them as work mules to rape with taxes, while our poor live like kings and queens popping out babies and driving brand new SUVs.

Even a small shift in IQ can dramatically increase the number of Retards and lower the rare gifted people. and two shifts lower reduces the number of gifted to just 1 million gifted people. These key gifted people are the ones who innovate society driving it forward. Without them, societies collapse. This means our nation could be fundamentally destroyed forever in just ten years with our current legal and illegal immigration policies and a welfare program that doesn't discourage births but instead rewards it with more dollahs and higher priority for free housing gibsmedat.

Solution? : How about drastically changing the lavish easy lifestyle that our poor and lazy get. Instead of Section 8 housing that places them in regular apartments, how about capsule mini-rooms just enough to survive. We continue to provide a middle class lifestyle but BETTER because they don't have to work – for the worst and laziest of us. If this continues America will indeed become an idiocracy. We have dropped from 90% of our births being Europanic in 1950 to less than 60% today. And that lower non-europanic life form has a higher violence and theft profile than a Europanic does, as well as being low IQ. These are called the Sociopathology – IQ relationship. Another key solution is to stop paying more for more babies. You get one basic welfare check for your family unit, a bit more if you are a dual parent family. No increases for having children but rather a bonus could be given out for every five years that someone does NOT have a child if they are within the fertile age of 12 to 35.

We have just a year or two left to switch the course this ship is on. It's a giant tanker, it turns slowly. Start now or go over the falls of IQ doom. How to do that? REWARD and RECOGNIZE our higher IQ students. Put them in special schools, not

INTEGRATED VIOLENT HELL SCHOOLS.

One county was recently sued to allow DIM students into AP classes because "thas raciss to keep muh chillin' out"

yehp.   Ah yehp.

Others studies showed that "0% of black students can read". It's frightful what has happened to our schools. Maybe the kids can't read because the dysgenic mutant teachers cannot read either. I'm not joking.

The Life-cycle of the Feminist Woman

Ahh the feminist woman. It all starts out so good for them. Refusing to find a quality mate they simply move to pure vanity and delusion and ego-centric narcissism from age 16-35. Instead of doing the things that would lead to a secure life in a marriage, they seek security from their career, or government welfare. Black girls as young as 15 know that they have to pop out 3 chillin' before high school ends to get on the section eight. That's hard for them, so many need a lag year or two at moms with all the babies until their number is called. For the career women, things are similar except they get to live in a world of huge numbers of single men, some starting out, others broken and divorced. But the basic math is two to one, and even the heffer three hundred pounders seem rife with bloat and I don't mean the fat, it's their egos.

Hyper inflated from endless male attentions, as males are playing their standard game mostly, a bit of riding the clutch then finding and picking one for marriage. But unbeknownst to them, that is NOT what women are doing. Women are in it for sport now. Marriage? that might come at 35 when they are ready for it post ten abortions, and five venereal diseases that weren't curable. Sadly the men have little clue the game has changed. If they find a fat, lazy and ugly enough one, she might settle for a younger marriage, almost instinctively knowing her days are numbered. But for most, its a grand party. It's a world that seems in endless celebration of them. and then one day… kaputsky. They suddenly age rapidly, estrogen goes down and wrinkles go up. It has fueled an entire economy of plastic surgery and frog face creams to keep them in the game just one more year.

If women are the "prize" why are they outnumbering Men 7-1

So as a male you really cannot imagine the life of these women. They don't have to study in college, they major in ridiculously absurd or easy majors, and unlike before they are not looking for their Mrs degree, no the workforce has been FORCED by government to give them make work jobs often in salaries MUCH higher than men. I was always shocked when teams I worked on got taken over by young women who were DIRECTORS and VPs with little experience and paid quite well. They were always disasters and wrecked the place. Well their life is one of shopping, feeding their egos, more shopping, and strutting and preening. It's a base behaviour except that it used to be to find a mate, now it has regressed into itself like a snake eating its own tail and struggling to digest not knowing why. Mobile slut apps serve merely to drive home that they are desireable and these women have no ability to decipher which are the men who want a relationship and which are Chads and Tyrones merely seeking to empty their loads for the evening. And it's quite odd that they cannot tell the difference or seem to actually distance themselves from future bethrothed. In the back of their minds they know the partying life ends with babies and marriage. Why do that before 40? There's still lotsa time.

College becomes a place to learn their skills and plow a few dozen men. But the post college decade fueled with enough money for a taxi to a fancy bar with cocktails and they take minus the tail home a lot of nights! It's good for cads, but gets boring even for men eventually. All of this going strong right past 30 as women start to get burned out or preggers and have to slowly start dropping out, or some dive into careers if they have some progress there, and think not of the happy life as a loving mom they have passed up.

The next stage is the larval stage as women find themselves between 32 and 45 and begin to realize that they are all partied out. After sex with 500 men, it really becomes just going through the motions orgasm or no orgasm. They lose their ability to pair bond, and with the endless abortia they lose their ability to deliver non-downy children and we ain't talking the laundry softener!

This is the confused stage for women. So they sign up for the marriage services, put on lotsa makeup, and make a desperate plea like a drowning victim likely to pull her savior down under as well. Don't be the man that falls into that trap. You need to seek out the rare plum, the 16-22 year old who can be swept out of the game before she is ruined from it. But it's quite hard. If you start looking post college it's already too late. You literally would have to start introducing yourself to dads with prospects for their 15 year old. Like that's likely to happen.

So now we come to the mid 40s and this is the desperation phase. But women, accustomed to a life of endless pandering and courting, seem a bit shocked when it slows down and the sideways eyes are coming from 70 year olds who think they might have a shot now.

In the desperation phase the one piece of advice for men is STAY AWAY this is not for you this is the used up refuse. And they will be quite clever in their depths to ensnare hapless betas. The smart inventive engineer entrepreneurs will stay far far away. They can only hope to snag a beta who has a boring cube slave job. Not to men in your forties, why do you put up with a boring cube slave job?

Finally it transitions to the chrysalis stage. Women get cats, too much plastic surgery, cakes of makeup, and walk fancy dogs. They find events to go to together like book clubs and wine nights and then as they truly age producing NOTHING for society that has coddled them and paid for them, they finally, if they have a shred of intellect, realize that the feminist dream is more like the feminist lie. But by then it's far too late.

Men keep chasing the 19-30 year olds continuing to re-inforce the cycle endlessly. Neither gender escapes unscathed. But for some men, those who walk away at 40 or 50 if they are able to do so pre-divorce rape, have some years to truly enjoy life if their work to death national mind set doesn't steal it all from them.

The Ice Age and Not Reproducing in Scarcity – It's In Our Genes

One of the most shocking things you experience when in Africa, the middle east, Asia, is how overpopulated it is. Or even if not so dense, they have reproduced far beyond what their resources can sustain. We call this R reproductive strategy. Have as many children as possible and hope some survive. This is in contrast to K reproductive strategy which is to have fewer children and invest in them, and then only have children when you have resources. This explains a lot of why the non Europanic races fall to welfare so quickly, they have children with abandon and without regard to what they can afford.

To pay for all this we have taxed the Europanics to such a degree that their K instincts kick in and they stop having children. They see society as unstable. This might be a lot of the reason why women seem "bitchy" and cold as times get more difficult, but loving and ready to settle down in the happy 50s and 60s, 80s, but not now.

It's in our very genes. It was THE survival mechanism during the ice age when the numbers of Europanics experienced a severe contraction. Some say less than 10,000 remained. To get through that limited children was key. But over in Africa it was still warm. The Africans never got the "stop the baby gene were out of food"

So now we endlessly send food to Africa, and they endlessly have more babies, requiring even more food aid to africa and on it's goes until Nigeria reaches a billion people.

Meanwhile, in the USA, the welfare-ites and the immigrant invaders – both peoples who never experienced the ice age and never had the K gene, reproduce as R strategy. For a long time we were told it was lack of access to birth control, but we'd easily and gladly donate enough, they still reproduce.

The tax flows away from the Europanics making it even worse. So they clutch in and have fewer babies, women feel like they MUST get a career and work to survive the new harder life and suddenly the population of the nation begins Kareeening (karening?) away from the producers to the slovenly class of misfits. We have to run budget deficits to pay for all the handouts and finally… our currency will die.

What can be done? Well it's genetic. So you have to cut off the food. You have to cut off the aid. You probably have to invest in science so you can turn on and off reproduction with a key. Our American free instincts don't like that. But we are facing extinction.

You could try financially to incentivise the welfare classes to get MORE money without children but I doubt it would work. Give them a bonus for turning off their reproduction at 16. If they chose a welfare path it stays off. If they marry or chose a productive life it gets turned on. Doesn't seem likely to work either.

No, we have spiteful mutants in our midst, the more we give them the more they hate us. Despise us. They are "kept down" because we are racist, not because of their own failures.

We are the Europanics, people made stronger from the cold and harsh environments which required planning for winter, food storage, and planning societies. We have innate feelings of charity and to take care of our own tribe that rarely exists in other races. The problem is invaders have impregnated into our tribal boundary and we cannot expulse them. Many Karen liberal women push to "feed the poor" and give them free housing. But they are not us. They are the cuckoos egg, now reborn and spread like a plague. We are just 50% of our tribe now but we have no way to split lest we get machine gunned down. It's an abysmal state. Just leave if you can but most cant. All trapped in a raping tax system that deprives us of prosperity and a fiat money system ever becoming more worthless as it's printed to pay for the cuckoos among us who have replaced us. But that's just a myth says Wikipedia and all the News outlets. Being replaced is a good thing says the Democrats. And the Re-blood-icans simply say they will work hard to stop it and then do nothing. So, our nation will die. It's just that simple. Our nation will die. We will be like Egypt and India, places where Europanics once existed, but destroyed by the rise of the spiteful mutants.

Educating the Spiteful Mutant Children – Fake Degrees Fake College Fake Jobs, Taxes for the Producers

You can't seem to have the choice to buy a house in a district that doesn't have a school. Cities get big development plans for 100 houses and it always includes schools. Always.

The school taxes are half your property taxes in most districts.

Well with the huge growth in the number of students, we need more schools they scream.

Except, when you look at whose playing at recess it's JimBumma and Kong, and Muhammed and Hesus, not david and kimberly and sarah.

> LOS ANGELES — Two years ago, a group of students and their teachers sued the state of California for doing a poor job teaching kids how to read — 53% of California third-graders did not meet state test standards that year, and scores have increased only incrementally since. On Thursday they won $53 million so that the state's lowest-performing schools have the resources to do better.

This is not my tribe. These are not my people. Yet pay for them I must. Somehow this is fair? "well you could choose to have kids" except, I wont go on welfare to afford them. because I'm not a spiteful mutant.

But it gets worse. The entire education is now utterly fake. Stories abound of the mutant children not being able to read at graduation. Worse, teachers are found not being able to read. No not the Europanic teachers, the Mutants who become teachers.

"Don Tell Me Muh Boo not AP" screamed one mother frantically. "Muh boo just as smart as those whitey kids it's just JUJU that they score better on tests, that's not fair, that's racist"

In Maplewood New Jersey the high school was considered segregated because although the student body is 40% Black only 20% of the students in AP classes are Black.

Black parents are convinced that their chillin are just as good as white chillin and only racism prevents them from attending the high IQ advanced placement classes.

Columbia high school in Maplewood, NJ, is being sued again for segregating students. This is the third such lawsuit over the last last 8 years. They settled with the Obama Administrations DOJ back in 2014, yet another lawsuits is pending. Back in 2014 when they settled with the Obama administration they eliminated testing requirements for AP classes. AP classes went from being 10% black to 20% Black , but this is still considered segregation. Since 40% of the students are Black they demand 40% of the students in AP classes should be Black.

Despite decades of effort and billions of dollars in funding, test scores for white, Asian American and wealthier students are much higher than those of their black, Latino and low-income peers. On computerized tests administered in the spring, for example, just 19 percent of African American students were proficient in math, compared with 73 percent of Asian American students.

Let's look at how the different races do on tests:

The IQs of racial groups in the United States based on all of the data presented here:

TIMSS stands for "Trends in International Math and Science Study", and gave a standard test to 42 countries on math and science. PISA stands for "Program for International Student Assessment" and gave a test for reading, math and science for 65 countries.

Time and time again blacks are found to have a borderline retarded IQ of 85 and Hispanics only do slightly better than that.

We can look at the worlds largest slums. They are all Black or Brown nations:

- **Khayelitsha** in Cape Town (**South Africa**): 400,000.
- **Kibera** in Nairobi (**Kenya**): 700,000.
- **Dharavi** in Mumbai (India): 1,000,000.
- **Neza** (Mexico): 1,200,000.
- Orangi Town in Karachi (Pakistan): 2,400,000.

In 2016, for example, the U.S. took in the most refugees from the Democratic Republic of the Congo (average IQ of 78), Syria (83), Burma/Myanmar (87), Iraq (87), and Somalia (68). (Mental retardation is defined as having an IQ of 70 or below.) These scores mean that, compared to immigrants from Japan (105), Taiwan (104), Italy (102), or Switzerland (101), these refugees will have higher rates of joblessness, incarceration, welfare use, and not obtaining a college degree.

Immigration data supports the theory. According to the Heritage Foundation, households headed by persons without a high school degree, on average, receive $46,582 in government benefits each year, but pay only $11,469 in taxes—a burden to taxpayers of $35,113 annually.

On the other hand, there are jobs and roles for the lower IQ peoples. And if they can be kept to 10% or less of the nation then they will follow the Europanic role models set for them. They will intrinsically be more violent and psychopathological as that is their genetics and brain structure. But it can be somewhat managed. Once this increases to 50% its game over for the society. It happened to Egypt. It happened to India. And now it's happening to the USA and Europe.

The big issue seems to be a misplaced leftist notion that all races are equal. While an argument that one race is superior to another seems to be not the point. More importantly there is a inventing high IQ race that forms productive society – the Europanics. There are also Asians, who have high IQ but are less inventive and are more easy to control in societies. Which is why they tend to be susceptible to communism.

Another misgiving is that these notions – recognizing the lessons of race, society and history – is somehow RACIST or done out of hatred for other races. Just the opposite, it is trying to use scientific realities and history to understand the doomsday scenario that happens if we do nothing. So staving off the genocide of our race and destruction of our society is "Racism"? Hardly. Racism implies an error. What is my error? There is no error. For example, if I say all black people have carrots for noses. Well that IS racism because it is an error. But if I say Blacks have an average IQ of 85 and much higher rates of crime and violence than Europanics in America, that isn't racism. Its science or fact or observation. The left has colluded and conjoined any talking about race as somehow Racism. It isn't true.

The big problem is that the USA has used the productive Europanic peoples as goats, work horses and worked them to death to the point that most can't afford to breed. Most of the middle class are leading frantic dismal trying to survive lives. And the big warning sign – a reproductive rate of 1.4 – is not recognized or addressed by the government. Instead we are stuck in a cycle of endless welfare-ism and endless warfare-ism with the federal reserve fiat money printing debasing the currency worse that 400AD Rome. What should we expect from this scenario? How do we address it? Do we seek a unified culture or a unified race?

Welfare use by first-generation immigrant households varies significantly by race as well, with the lowest rates among Asians and whites, and the highest rates among those from Central America, Mexico, the Caribbean, and Africa:

Such welfare use continues even after immigrants are well-established. In come cases, it actually increases before it goes slightly down

Remember in these studies "Natives" often includes black and brown races.

We need to set up the reproductive strategies so that the middle class CAN afford children and turn DOWN the handouts so that the brown races cannot do well and don't want children on welfare. For example, cut the payola for having more children on welfare while offering a bonus for not having children every three years. If they will go insane for the 40" tv at walmart, think how crazy they might get to have a $2000 check.

America has a hard work ethic culture that came from the Puritans and Protestants and Settlers. The problem is that blacks do not share in it. A large reason for this is the rewards system is very anti intellectual in America. Become an engineer and you'll get watered down middle class wages for busting your ass because of the 5 million h-1b savages here who have take your jobs. Become a rapper and you'll get millions for barking like a dog. Or become a sportster and again, lavished with millions. Should you try to be a writer or a talking head on TV? Most writers will never be successful while the dumb TV heads get millions each year. So that reward-outcome shows a completely screwed up society and there's just no fixing it in the short term. But a lot of the distortions COME from the fiat currency and Fed Central banking system where they can flood sectors selectively with dollars. Cities can demand taxes on property (that should be very illegal! it's against the constitution! It's against the foundation of capitalism!) and then decide to hand a Billion dollar brand new play stadium to billionaires so that their players can play and still have millions left over to pay them tremendously. And for many many years, you could not get cable tv without paying your tithe to the sport monkies. It was a racket. A shakedown. And finally that's crumbling.

So everyone who argues against the issue of preserving the founding people of a country always take the extreme position. That our goal must be eradication of all races from the planet. Or something nuts like that. Instead, all we are talking about is wanting to stand AGAINST THE GENOCIDE OF OUR PEOPLE AND AGAINST THE EXTERMINATION OF OUR NATION. The USA simply isn't viable financially with a population of 60% brown people of whom HALF are on the gibsMeDAT system. Already as is we are flying headlong into bankruptcy and default at a rate of 1,500,000,000,000 a year. Thats a lot! The interest is rising above 600 billion dollars a year on our budget. That's a lot! This is ALREADY crisis mode. But it's never talked about. That makes everyone else a complete imbecile as far as I'm concerned.

Meanwhile the Demothugs and the left push for MORE MORE BROWN PEOPLE. Endless open borders, ending ice, black thugs matter, and RACISM in government and Education – dumb blacks getting into harvard, blacks and hispanics getting government freebies and priorities on contracts, it's all madness. All of that should be stopped immediately. But it wont be.

Sadly our nation will die and our people will be extinguished. It's quite horrible. And it appears there's nothing that can be done about it. The USA will be flushed down the toilet bowl of History just like Egypt and India. Our new brown people will be non-productive and the middle class will revert to huts and shit in the streets. It's already happening in California.

So what to do? Well we write. We talk. We try to wake people up. But we get called RACIST because our brains function and we can look at simple unimpeachable facts and call that reality and truth. When you are striving to save your entire nation, the cries of Racism no longer sting. When you are saving billions of your people yet to be born, the cries of Fascist no longer hurt. We see the history behind us, after us, and our current situation clearly. Race does matter and it must be controlled. Our DYSGENIC nation cannot continue on this course and survive or we will become a GHETTO NATION.

"Ai is not too dumb to teach" said Jessica Jones, a black teacher who recently flunked the teaching test. But sadly only 26% of blacks can pass it. Hispanics don't do much better with only 40% able to pass the simple test.

"This is WHITEWASHING, THIS IS RACIST" screamed a teacher who had flunked it a second time.

But the questions are very simple.

"If a man can eat two apples a day, how many days does it take for him to eat ten apples"

"That's RACISS too!" screamed Jessica- "Everyone knows apples are white people food"

State data shows Borges is one of 60% of Hispanic examinees who failed the GK math test last year. While black examinees also experienced disproportionately high failure rates with 74% flunking the test during the same time frame. However, of Caucasian examinees who took the same test, 43% failed, leaving the majority passing the test last year.

Lee County's school district hiring boss, Dr. Angela Pruitt, started studying the racial and gender breakdown of its own teachers taking the exam because so many were repeatedly failing it.

"It's a concern," she said. "If we're struggling to get recruitment in minority categories than that makes recruitment that much harder," she said. Pruitt is also calling on the state to offer more alternatives to people who would like to teach in Florida instead of putting so much emphasis on the FTCE exam as a prerequisite to teach.

When the test was revised, failures increased

In 2015, portions of the tests were revised and made more difficult. According to the FLDOE which oversees the tests, the tests were made more rigorous to better align with more rigorous student tests.

But two years ago, Investigative reporter Katie LaGrone discovered that immediately after those revisions were implemented, failure rates began to increase dramatically with failures on some sections of the test increasing by 30%.

Over the past two years, LaGrone has detailed how the increase in failures on the test has resulted in statewide fallout at virtually every level of Florida's education system. Some of the fallout she's reported include:

- More than 1,000 teachers were terminated this past summer despite having records of being effective or highly effective teachers.
• already struggling to fill empty classrooms have been forced to fill more positions or higher long-term substitutes to fill those positions.
• College of Education programs have seen a decrease in enrollment and increase in the length of time it takes students to graduate.

The kids aren't doing better either.

> Three of four African-American boys in California classrooms failed to meet reading and writing standards on the most recent round of testing, according to data obtained from the state Department of Education and analyzed by CALmatters. The reading data is sobering. As early as fourth grade, for example, nearly 80 percent of black boys failed to meet state reading standards.

On the 2015 National Assessment of Educational Progress, only 18 percent of African-American fourth-graders were proficient in reading and only 19 percent scored as proficient in math, according to an analysis by the U.S. Chamber of Commerce Foundation released Friday. The eighth-grade numbers were even worse, with only 16 percent of African-American students proficient in reading and 13 percent proficient in math.

African-American students were lagging far behind their white classmates in every measure of academic success: grade-point average, standardized test scores, and enrollment in advanced-

placement courses. On average, black students earned a 1.9 GPA while their white counterparts held down an average of 3.45. Other indicators were equally dismal. It made no sense.
When these depressing statistics were published in a high school newspaper in mid-1997, black parents were troubled by the news and upset that the newspaper had exposed the problem in such a public way. Seeking guidance, one parent called a prominent authority on minority academic achievement.UC Berkeley Anthropology Professor John Ogbu had spent decades studying how the members of different ethnic groups perform academically.

He'd studied student coping strategies at inner-city schools in Washington, DC. He'd looked at African Americans and Latinos in Oakland and Stockton and examined how they compare to racial and ethnic minorities in India, Israel, Japan, New Zealand, and Britain. His research often focused on why some groups are more successful than others.But Ogbu couldn't help his caller. He explained that he was a researcher — not an educator — and that he had no ideas about how to increase the academic performance of students in a district he hadn't yet studied. A few weeks later, he got his chance. A group of parents hungry for solutions convinced the school district to join with them and formally invite the black anthropologist to visit Shaker Heights. Their discussions prompted Ogbu to propose a research project to figure out just what was happening. The district agreed to finance the study, and parents offered him unlimited access to their children and their homes.

The professor and his research assistant moved to Shaker Heights for nine months in mid-1997. They reviewed data and test scores. The team observed 110 different classes, from kindergarten all the way through high school. They conducted exhaustive interviews with school personnel, black parents, and students. Their project yielded an unexpected conclusion: It wasn't socioeconomics, school funding, or racism, that accounted for the students' poor academic performance; it was their own attitudes, and those of their parents.

Ogbu concluded that the average black student in Shaker Heights put little effort into schoolwork and was part of a peer culture that looked down on academic success as "acting white."

Citing the fact that an outsized percentage of black and Hispanic candidates were failing the test, members of the New York state Board of Regents plans to adopt a task force's recommendation to eliminate the literacy exam, known as the Academic Literacy Skills Test, given to prospective teachers.

In Detroit, black parents gathered together to sue the teachers for failure. Sadly the failure is in their own genetics. In the end the issue is not to fix the education, but to fix the jobs that these people are vying for. A few will be able to be come doctors, lawyers, engineers. But very few. Some will be great thinkers like Sowell. But the bell curve tells a difficult story.

The numbers of the 120+ IQ blacks is thousands of times rarer than for Europanic men. Instead these need to be identified early and put on that track, but for the rest, basic business training basic trades and even basic burden work should be the coursework. Training in showing up for work on time and the value of a hard days work and a simple life. All our efforts of pushing them into college high brained programs only makes them decry RACISM when their outcomes don't match those of the High IQ Europanic people around them. And now that same misuse of Egalitarianism and misunderstanding is fomenting violence in America, ANGER that they do not have the paths to prosperity opened to them. So time and time again, tests to become firemen, police officers, government workers are all removed. The once high standards for civil service are forgotten. And our nation rots out of fear of offense. A stinking deep rot. Walk the streets of Detroit and you can smell it.

So the final stage is to have fake college spots for these low brained mutants, easy majors like race studies or lesbian weaving, and then they graduate and get fake jobs which companies take on as pure overhead, waste, just to not be sued for not hiring enough of the mutants in their midst.

Now so many dumb kids go to college that colleges are mostly fake outside the top tier. Its just one big part and a huge pile of debt for dumb kids. "I IS A COLLEGE GRADURATE" Colleges have degraded because of the mutants so much, with total nutters like Evergreen threatening their white teachers, high school mutants beating up and nearly killing their teachers, general mayhem in the halls, it's basically destroyed education for Europanics. A Europanic mother who sends her children to these horror halls should be charged with child abuse.

What to do? Have everything be done by software. Pre-programmed courses of study from 1 to 100. You have to pass the level to move forward. Enough of mutant children who are at level 2 at age 17 with Europanic children at level 250 at age 12. And the penalty for these Atlanta teachers who cheat the tests? Public whipping. Nothing less.

Better yet, home school the kids with these same well developed programs. Ah but you still have to pay that education tax on your property. If you home school or have no kids you should be exempt. Because we no longer have kids. So its just flat out RAPE of our race, and transferring resources to the dumb mutants who are just pretending to be educated. It's like Charleston Heston in Planet of the Apes – "It's a MADHOUSE, A MADHOUSE"

Genome Exhaustion After Being Conquered: Why Some Races Seem Terrible

This is one of those controversial "Racist" topics that gets lefty chicks who don't wear bras (the only good thing about lefty chics, er at least for that year until they start to sag, you have to find those with the perky tangerines not the grapefruits or it will go south fast!). OK now that we've started off on an atrocious note, let's get serious.

Let's take a hypothetical race called the Loserheim. The Winnerheim are smarter and stronger than the Loserheim, but for a time, as long as they were separate, the Loserheim seemed to do quite well. Then one day they go to war.

All of Loserheim's smartest and strongest and most alpha men end up dead. What's left is the sniveling hiding cowards. The industrious women simply declare their loyalty and love for Winnerheim men and quickly blend into the gene pool. So what's left in Loserheim? Well the spiteful mutants basically. Worse, the yoke of enslavement or subservience continues to weed out all the upshoots of tougher braver men. Over time all thats left is an exhausted race.

It reminds me of my apple tree and the Texas heat. It did fine for several years, but one year it got god awful hot. The tree looked dead after. When spring came, only a few new shoots tried to poke out from the trunk and start anew, all the taller branches were dead.

That's genetics. Now let's take a look at some of the actual races and how they fit into this. After world war II Americans mostly returned home unscathed. The Japanese lost a lot of their strongest men, but not all. They would become a somewhat meak race thereafter which doesn't resemble at all the Meiji and Shogunate eras. Now look at Germany. Germany was ravaged to the GROUND and BURNT DOWN. Dresden was firebombed and 200,000 innocent civilians were burnt to a crisp by the Americans. But even worse, after the war, all the german men who fought were rounded up and put into starvation cages (see the book on the front page – Hellstorm). When wives tried to bring them food, they were pushed away. Morgantheu literally authorized the complete raping of Germany, removing all their farm and industrial equipment. It was a race utterly sacked and destroyed.

But yes, over a time German did rebuild. But not as fast as the Japanese. And the communist sector less so – breeding the LEAST and most SNIVELING and CONNIVING of men. That's what communism forces you into. They get the rewards. Communism is the ultimate goal of all spiteful mutants. You might call them Democrats today. But the way it works is over time there is less and less spoils to feed off of and then things just get worse and worse until a fatigue sets into the population and everything just starts going really slow – they became pickled in the 1950s age. When the wall came down and Germany re-united east Germany was like a fun frolic to a museum. In east Prenzlauerberg (the east side of Berlin) they had these almost disney like crossing lamps with men in little hats. How quaint people thought, not realizing it was all evidence of a society destroyed.

The american indians, another loser in a war, similary went through decades of bloodshed constantly losing their fierce warriors. Finally the death march called the trail of tears was one final sorting. Well at least Indians should technically be good at long marches. Their fighting spirit left them. Their strongest alpha males gone, and welfare put upon them to destroy selective breeding processes that would have revived them, they are a half dead race. But still, strong shoots. The independent tribes and especially their casinos suddenly sprung up a strong race of entrepreneurs who become ever more financially savy and strong. But back on the reservations and welfare land, its a dismal doomsville.

Now let's go to the source of Amerinds who still remain in south America and central America. Tough strong hard working industrious people. Lively with a strong spirit. There is NO WELFARE in their nations except perhaps some basic medical system. So they must produce to survive. When the spanish left Guatemala their beautiful churches in Antigua collapsed from a huge earthquake. The Amerinds simply looked on unable to fathom how to reconstruct them. And that is how they remain today. They are a industrious people, but do not match the Europanics or East Asian in IQ and mathematics which are pre-requisites to perform the complex architecture and construction of a cathedral. Even KNOWING the original design, they were at a loss to repair them.

The american blacks were rousted and captured by stronger tribes. They were already at a disadvantage. Next the slave ships took another tool as those who fought back were thrown off the boat. Add to that a hundred years of killing and crushing the upstarts who fought back and you again get an exhausted race. Which again would have bounced back were it not for the welfare system ending all selective breeding. Are there great black people. Of course. Many of my heroes are black. Thomas Sowell senior fellow at he Hoover institute at Stanford dispelled many of the myths blacks clung to. Musically there are too many to name. Nina Simone is enough to redeem the entire race. But sadly, the welfare system bred the worst of the lot becoming ever worser. Gangsterism, Thuggy-ism, accosted with an educational system that just looked the other way as it became ever more communist and ensuring equal outcomes for brainiacs and savages alike. The entire American education system is at this point utterly destroyed and any sane parent who leaves their child there should be charged with abuse. It's where the commies nestle. A combined calcification of shitty single mothers who are too lazy to raise their own children and lazy women who want jobs to not teach. But that is another story.

Occasionally I'll meet an immigrant from Ethiopa. They are polite and erudite, and even bagging groceries seem to have that lost and dead american spirit of making something of themselves. And with affirmative action, another death poison from the commies, many are getting back into regular life, even if it's only a charade of working, get decent pay, and start to shake off the welfare root strangling them. But it's not enough. The gene pool is so thoroughly wrecked their proclivity towards crime and rejection of learning and hard work (don't even think Pioneer spirit here) is overwhelming. Until welfare reform happens it will remain so.

But even WITHOUT the slave trade Africa was behind. African brains are smaller and lower IQ than Europanics. They lack the inventiveness. So do Asians. who can outperform Europanics on math. Amerinds have higher IQs than Hispanics, but seem also to have much higher incidences of psychopathology. (see Richard Lynn's seminole book, an excerpt of which can be read here https://www.amren.com/news/2008/08/race_and_psycho/)

Once again the same pattern is repeated. When the colonial powers left Africa to allow them to set their own path, very quickly things began to break and fall into disrepair. In Liberia the British sewer systems broke and people began to relieve themselves on the beaches. Within a few years any hope of having a tourist trade to visit perfect gleaming white sands was gone forever. Some nations convert their UN and Global handout money to bring in teams of Europanics to work the OIL refineries and sewage systems.

It works for a time. Eventually they will succumb to financial collapse and of their own means they will not be able to maintain them.

Eventually they will revert to what they are capable of due to their genetics. This uplifting is not only pointless but destructive. Shipping them 50 million used American t-shirts every year destroyed their clothing industries. Shipping them 500 million tons of food every year destroys their incentives to farm. It's welfare but called relief. Worse, as they breed endlessly with R reproductive strategy (without regard for sustaining their children) they run out of resources. This is called drought and famine. Oh we must do something. Sadly we have done far too much. Better that we walk away. Oh we must import refugees their nations are at war. Their nations are always at war and they bring that waring with them. We have to stop confusing NATURAL STATE from something that is "climate change" or temporary. Somalia no longer has a government and has descended into piratism, Congo nearly the same. There are genocidal extinction wars between the races. Well, you can't claim Europanics are that much better, we are bitter war like savages shackled temporarily by the atomic bomb. We have a bitter history of a 1000 years of warring among ourselves over petty differences.

So some of the mysteries of why some races have different strenghts and weaknesses in different areas isn't so hard to ponder. Consider racial exhaustion in the genotype as a primary but penultimate consideration on top of the million years of evolution. The IQ genes do not necessarily map to the psychopathology genes do not map to the athletic sprinter genes or the ability to see in bright sunlight across vast lands covered in white snow (the blue eyes genes). They are all different branches of the genome and can become increased or decreased by the environment. And the deadliest things in the environment are communism, feminism, and welfare.

Where are the Egyptians? Total Dysgenic Displacement of a Nation is the future the USA and Europe Faces

Once upon a time, three thousand years ago, Egyptians were proud white people. Slightly tanned middle eastern like one might have found in Pompei or southern Italy. But Caucasian non the less. And recent genetic testing of mummies has proven it now beyond any question.*(see article below) While Awasi tried to suppress the results (himself not very white) the results were leaked and are now accepted. And it matches with their history and drawings. They were a white race. And they flourished.

Have you visited Egypt recently? It's a filthy pit of brown people honking horns, cutting chicken heads off in the streets, a far cry from the beautiful temples that the Caucasians built. How did this happen?

Egypt was the first well known nation to fall to Dysgenics – that is their genetic stock literally had gotten contaminated and polluted by lesser races to the degree that there was nothing left of the original people. Whether this involved direct mating with Nubian slaves or simply being out-reproduced, they were replaced. A civilization that lasted six thousand years is now no more.

What you will find time and again is that Caucasians have a K reproductive strategy – high investment in children, and less willingness to reproduce in tough times to bring their population down to match resources. This is fine until a R reproductive (reproduce like rabbits always with no regard for resources or ability to care for children) race moves in. Then gradually over time by sheer reproductive will, the K race is replaced. This is why homelands MUST be protected and separated from invading races. yet this is precisely what is happening to the USA and

Europe today.

The USA is already massively overcrowded and running low on key resources like water, food, and definitely Highways for all those cars. So the native Caucasian population FEELS this stress and begins to pull back from families and making babies. This is what a K Reproductive species do. This includes Asians as well, and studying the statistics one could argue that they are even MORE likely to halt reproduction in response to crowding and stress – that is the case in Japan today. Have you seen the sardine can subways of Tokyo? They have Human PUSHERS to force more people on. Do you feel like you need more kids when that is happening? Heck no!

Nertiti's Bust Clearly Shows Caucasian Features – Born 1370 BC

America's invasion by central Americans, Africans, and African welfare breeding programs has already radically reduced the Europanic population of the USA from 91% in 1960 to 55% today in 2019. By 2030-2040, Europanics with be the minority race, and there simply won't be a large enough productive tax base to pay for the welfare and social security and disability (90% of blacks qualify as low IQ individuals). What happens then? That's only 15 years from now!

As Japan's population pulls back, many of their small towns in the country are dying out. But soon one would expect teams of hipsters and bohos to go HEY let's take that town and start farming its all FREE! Still the draw of the congested cities jobs and money pulls strong.

Let us mourn the death of the Egyptians. As nation after nation falls to a dysgenic invasion we must ask ourselves the question – Is my country next?

Modern "Egyptians" are a different people than the pyramid builders

The team sampled 151 mummified individuals from the archaeological site of Abusir el-Meleq, along the Nile River in Middle Egypt, from two anthropological collections hosted and curated at the University of Tübingen and the Felix von Luschan Skull Collection at the Museum of Prehistory of the Staatliche Museen zu Berlin, Stiftung Preussicher Kulturbesitz.

In total, the authors recovered partial genomes from 90 individuals, and genome-wide datasets from three individuals. They were able to use the data gathered to test previous hypotheses drawn from archaeological and historical data, and from studies of modern DNA.

"In particular, we were interested in looking at changes and continuities in the genetic makeup of the ancient inhabitants of Abusir el-Meleq," said Alexander Peltzer, one of the lead authors of the study from the University of Tübingen.

The team wanted to determine if the investigated ancient populations were affected at the genetic level by foreign conquest and domination during the time period under study, and compared these populations to modern Egyptian comparative populations.

"There is literary and archaeological evidence for foreign influence at the site, including the presence of individuals with Greek and Latin names and the use of foreign material culture," said co-author W. Paul van Pelt from Cambridge's Division of Archaeology. "However, neither of these provides direct evidence for the presence of foreigners or of individuals with a migration background, because many markers of Greek and Roman identity became 'status symbols' and were adopted by natives and foreigners alike. The combined use of artefacts, textual evidence and ancient DNA data allows a more holistic study of past identities and cultural exchange or 'entanglement'."

The study found that the inhabitants of Absur el-Meleq were most closely related to ancient populations in the Levant, and were also closely related to Neolithic populations from the Anatolian Peninsula and Europe. "The genetics of the Abusir el-Meleq community did not undergo any major shifts during the 1,300 year timespan we studied, suggesting that the population remained genetically relatively unaffected by foreign conquest and rule," said Wolfgang Haak, group leader at the Max Planck Institute for the Science of Human History, and a co-author of the paper.

The data shows that modern Egyptians share approximately 8% more ancestry on the nuclear level with sub-Saharan African populations than the inhabitants of Abusir el-Meleq, suggesting that an increase in sub-Saharan African gene flow into Egypt occurred within the last 2,000 years. Possible causal factors may have been improved mobility down the Nile River, increased long-distance trade between sub-Saharan Africa and Egypt, and the trans-Saharan slave trade that began approximately 1,300 years ago.

Reference:
Verena J. Schuenemann et al. 'Ancient Egyptian mummy genomes suggest an increase of Sub-Saharan African ancestry in post-Roman periods.' Nature Communications (2017). DOI: 10.1038/ncomms15694

The Dysgenic Effect of Divorce Rape

Smart men quickly realize the dangers of marriage or even sex in the new Feminazi me-too empowered women world. It's a losing game for men. Divorce courts routinely take 75% of mens assets even retirement savings and hand them over to women. Then demand 75% of your salary be handed over as well. Search Youtube for Dave Foley if you think that's not true. While it's worse in the Mega-Feminazi demothug cities, it's pretty much everywhere unless you live in Butte.

But this is having a radical effect on the quality of our babies. Welfare hoodlums who sell the tooth fall out powder at night have LOTS of Babies. Dumb beta males who just don't know better or think better have LOTS of Babies. Alpha Chads and Tyrones who are generally dumb as a stump have LOTS of babies. But smart people? Not so much.

This is the inverse of Darwin. Hence it's an artificial dysgenic situation caused by government policy. and that policy is the divorce rape of the male backed up by 2 shots of free housing and money for life if that falls through.

More and more smart men are stepping away from the work-exhaust-enslaved treadmill and beginning to think of working for themselves, taking care of themselves and waiting out the 500 year madness we are embarking upon until society fizzles out and changes or gets invaded by the Chinee or Hijab people.

Of course, we won't see a population decrease, that's what immigration is for, to hide that shocking facts so it's not quite so obvious. Population keeps going up, but it's not us who are having the children it is the other.

The other aren't bad, but certainly not the tough pioneer stock that founded this nation nor the inventive stock that gave us our political thought and inventions which basically is all of modern society. But if that government is now so corrupted as to destroy the nation, then it needs to go. And go it will. A new age of barbarism, a road warrior future for failed lands is what is ahead of us. First the welfare collapse and the cannibalism. Then when we are exhausted the replacement gene pattern from China or Arabia will come in and take over. One will do it en mass with millions, the other simply breeds away on welfare in the shadows creating a geometric growth in their babies.

Divorce rape horror won't ever change or be reformed by courts. Women have the good life now. One foolish man getting married and they get to smile inside, another sucker taken, their life will now be funded forever, unless of course they drive him to suicide. So they have to be careful only to inflict massive amounts of torture to make him give up, like the black widow biting her mate with just enough poison so he can continue the mating act, but not so much that he can ever get away. That's the modern trap.

There is an answer. Vasectomy, no co-habitating with women, and for some, full monk mode. Men are on strike. The good ones will come back when the laws change. Until then, invest in video game stocks and electronic sex doll wifus, cause men will need a replacement.

And as android wives get smarter and more mobile, this may seem like a good situation for both sexes, until the women wake up at 40 and whine "where are all the good men" well ladies you divorce raped them to exhaustion then you ME-TOO'd them in the dating game until they were scared as crickets to even go near you. And you wonder where the men are. for shame.

Life on the Tax Iceberg... Soon it will tip over

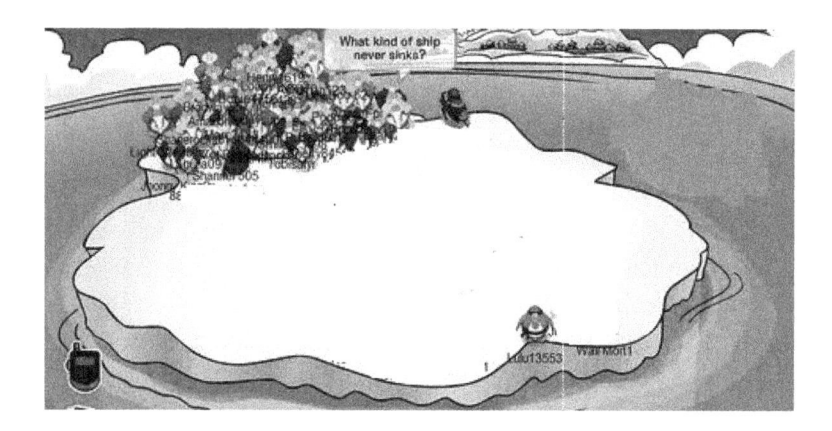

So imagine you are a sole productive worker on one side of an iceberg. A thin one that's floating on top of the water. Near the center on one side are 20 spiteful mutants. They are net tax receivers. They have set up their lives to use other peoples money.

Your weight opposes them. So you have to slink out to the far side. If you don't balance their weight it will tip over.

You didn't have any children because of the divorce rape courts and the high taxes placed on you make it impossible. The property taxes are particularly painful. Education taxes you pay through your property taxes pay for the spiteful mutant's children to get educated. Many just snuck into the country to get that freebee – it's not offered in Guatemala or Nicaragua. So you've been utterly exhausted. But they keep having more and more children, the more children they have the more money they get!

You look back, and there are now 50 spiteful mutants. Their side begins to sink down. What happens? You have no choice but to go to the extreme edge of the iceberg lest everyone die.

And this is precisely what is happening with our tax system, as well as our invisible tax system – inflation. Every years wages don't rise, pensions disappear for regular working folk, and you get pushed further and further to the edge of the iceberg.

As the percentage of the population of spiteful mutants rises, the weight and pressure on the producers will increase. They will literally get squeezed for more and more.

When we look at the states which have fallen to demothugs we see that they have huge populations of invaders and other spiteful mutants. This is by design. This is how they rule ya. The same is true for cities. If you put the Asians and Europanics on one side of the iceberg and the dysgenics and spiteful mutants on the other, ask yourself will this tip over. All the failed cities show this is the case. And now we have moved up from cities to failed states.

OK it's 2035. The government has overspent so the deficit is 100 trillion. The social security trust is insolvent. What to do? Declare the deficit expunged and simply start over printing more dollars. Inflation soars to 20% a year and taxes keep going up.

At this point the ice berg has flipped. clinging to the edge of one side as the spiteful mutant population increases and increases, finally you say screw this. and you let go and dive into the ocean. Shortly thereafter all the mutants pile into the ocean as well, their parasitic host now gone.

What does this mean in real terms for the USA? Food shortages. Housing shortages. People living 10 to a room without heat or water. No people fixing things because that takes producers. The adult babies and welfare queens will find their checks don't pay for very much anymore. And the productive class? Well they will be somewhere else, dispersed through other countries which don't have welfare and don't have property taxes. America is no longer the place to be if you want to be successful and it's certainly not the place to be retired.

Sadly America was successful because it was free. But we weren't free because of the huge taxation on everything. So our success has gone. Maybe Mehico is better now. Low taxes, and a bit of violent cartel murdering here and there. Eh, still might be better than the USA. Or a beachy island in the Phillipines like Siargaw. Sure Duterte hates Americans, but at least they have coconuts. Columbia is booming and the coke is abundant, so thats a good place to launch a startup company. Keeps you going through those long nights of coding. Or maybe dying and emptying out Portugal, now further along in the no births collapse than the USA, rents in the countryside small towns are dirt cheap. And they have the most delicious pastries there! No in this new digital work from Anywhere age, America is no longer the be all and end all place, and certainly the megalopilis Chicago and New York are just old dinosaurs decaying were it not for their financial and banking hubs there they would probably blow away like sand in the wind.

2035 is only fifteen years away. Think this isn't going to happen? Maybe they can cobble together 5 more years. But they would have had to have changed course today, right now. Instead they are printing 8 trillion to pay for a virus.

The lower middle class will become the poor. the middle middle class will become the poor. And only the upper middle class will carry on any semblance of normal American life. The old movies and films of what life used to be will be deleted.

If we froze welfare payola today and ended free section 8 housing, abolished property taxes and education taxes, we might have a chance. But that never will happen.

100 more people are now on the other side of the iceberg. Your fingers cling to the edge as you hang off one side trying to balance their weight. It's impossible. Because we thought we could manage 10 million on welfare and disability somehow we

thought we could manage half our working population on welfare and disability. The America where everyone worked hard is over. There aren't any solutions any more. Sadly its the meat grinder for most of us. Why? The rich politicos were happy eating lobster and driving bugattis. They were quite happy with skimming riches off the top. The Re-blood-lickins didn't accomplish even the first tiny steps when they were in power. Build the wall they cheer. Yes, a wall with huge gaps, and no machine guns on the other side. My nation is dying and I've made my peace with that.

The truth is we've been replaced. The hard working can do pioneer spirit has been replaced with gibs-me-dat (free money). Let me relate a story from real life. For years I'd take my pool leaf rakes and get the nets replaced each year. Then my local pool store got replaced by a chain, then the old employees replaced by millenials. I pluked the leaf rake on the counter. "I need to replace the net" pointing to the big hole in it. A few minutes later, a low IQ employee returned with another complete leaf rake, a crappy one, for $40 bucks. "No" I replied " I just want it re-netted". "No, we are millennials, we don't know how to do things" replied the vacuous eyed minimum waged air breather. Ok they only said "Uh... we don't do that" but you get the message. In truth at least they were showing up for work. A notch above the welfare and disability queens, the hispanicos whos "husbands" work for cash mowing lawns while the single wives get free housing and checks, better than the blacks who say they have a twinge in their backs and stop working at 20 if they ever worked at all, better than the black and hispanic women who have babies just to get on the dole, better than the pinko commie simp men who claim to have ADHD and sip lattes all day, better than the feminists who get fraud degrees then take jobs from men but do no work at all and can't be fired because companies are afraid. No, these sad vessels were the best of what's coming.

It can't be that bad you say. They thought the same thing about Detroit. But when the fires and riots broke out the productive fled the city and now its just zombies on welfare. It's the same at the country level, the only thing that has kept most Americans here is that most other nations are worse. That won't be true in ten years. It really isn't true now.

What kind of ship never sinks? a Dictatorship!

The New Baby Crisis

The American era has established a global maritime security, so free long range trade has been possible.

America's future is to withdraw from the world as our reach has to be reduced and we set up one to one relationships with other favored nation. That is NOT China. To one degree or another. no other nation will continue as a power except America. We are uniquely situated to be a self sufficient empire. The problem is, our financial debt is about to come crashing down. What then becoes of America?

There are demographic disasters in nearly every other country (except France and Australia). But more than numbers, it's also the QUALITY of the people. We have been on a program of replacing our citizens in the two worst way – breeding our welfare minions endlessly, and illegal invaders from third world nations without the high IQ breeding stock to replenish our nation.

So while it may appear by the simple numbers that America's demographic destiny is no big problem, its a lot more to accomplish than simply have other nations children. The new populations will lack several aspects of American can do high IQ make it happen phenotype. Instead it's more likely to be welfare scamming, a bit lazy, and certainly not that bright peoples. And now they are us. Because every president thinks there's endless time to fix things. But there isn't.

So first thing to recognize is our TOTAL fertility rate has dropped from 2.1 a decade ago to 1.7. That's a demographic disaster. If we use RACE as a PROXY for spiteful mutant (non productive slag) – yes, it's not quite a tautology but it's close – we see that of the two races which produce new productivity – Europanics and Asians (white is a racist term) – reproduction rates have slipped to 1.6 and 1.5 respectively. That means a population reduction of FIFTY PERCENT in FIFTY years. Very quickly the welfare needs of the many will overrun the tax production of the few, or the one. We don't have to drop in productive population that much before we go into negative tailspin, one could argue that we already have. Hence the national debt. This can only accelerate, the cuts to the spending would be so massive to bring our economic future under control congress would never approve it. Going from a Trillion dollar budget to 300 billion. Our defense budget is over 700 billion. So instead they go with continue to inflate and continue to print money.

That was an ok strategy for the short term. But the huge costs of the covid bailout, and again the fed taking FOUR TRILLION dollars in bad bonds and loans and CDOs onto its balance sheet to prop up the bankers who made bad loans (can you say fracking) is a serious issue. They will simply deny inflation and deny interest rates from rising. Hmm. So they are forcing a made up non-market driven price for dollars. It's weird. No one really knows. It's like keeping the cap on a bottle you keep pumping with more air, eventually something isa gonna BLOW! Current estimates put it at 2035. But the reality is the first hiccups of this impossible monetary policy will bite within 10 years. Trump will be long gone by then, House Pelosi will have to fix it. Yah right like that's going to happen.

There is a winning strategy in that if we can bide our time and be a bit frugal and massively productive and efficient just a bit longer, we will see the other houses burst first. We then can go

OH this ain't good. And pretty soon the globalist and demothug concept of population replacement to deal with low birth will need a good trouncing. There is still a strategy we can take. End birthright citizenship, establish e-verify, and tax the hell out of invaders if we can't send them home. Make it a much more difficult proposition so they have to MATCH the hearty German Irish and Italians who came here in the industrial boom of last century. At that point it matters not if they come because they will not be spiteful mutants sucking off freebies but converted to real productive members of society with a bit of thuggin on the side. Yes you can never escape the differences in racial psychopathology.

But that could be managed if you manage the percent of population – say 20% that is limited to the more psychopathological races. Blacks have already gobbled up 14% of that so there's only 6% for all the hispanics to fit into or about 20 million. That means 60 million hispanics need to leave. Sorry that's the equation for a productive cash positive nation. It's grim but it's reality. Or we just accept the murder and rape levels of Nigeria and Brazil and call that the new normal. That's the more likely end game, with more Europanic enclaves and more racial separation getting faught by demothug seeding with Section 8 housing so that there can be no escape from rape and murder by the productive races. How long will we put up with that. Forever, merely mentioning the word race has banned this book forever.

Race and Crime:

Since there is no Hispanic category in the FBI's Uniform Crime Reports and approximately 93 percent of Hispanics identify themselves, or are identified by law enforcement officers, as white, most arrests of Hispanics are added to white violent crime rates.

"The result is that the violent crime rates for whites are inflated and the black rates are deflated in these studies," says Steffensmeier.

When the researchers adjusted for the Hispanic effect, there was little overall change in the black percentage of violent crime.

Using arrest statistics from 1980 to 2008 in California and New York, two states that include a Hispanic category, the recalculated national figures indicated that the black percentage of assault increased slightly from 42 percent to 44 percent and homicide increased from 57 percent to 65 percent. There was a small decline in robbery, from 57 percent to 54 percent.

"It is the case that violent crime rates are lower today for blacks, as they also are for other race groupings, but the black percentage of violent crime is about the same today as in 1980," says Steffensmeier.

So as we look at these "official" crime rates by race, which are already abhorrently skewed, the reality is most likely the Europanic crime rate is 50% less and the black and hispanic are 50% higher. Ok, let's use the fake statistics that they tried to make the other races look better. It's still a total shit-show for non-asian non-europanics.

There are 4.6 times as many Europanics as blacks according to official 2016 numbers. So let's multiple the black murder rate to be able to compare it to the Europanic numbers and we get:

Black 20,217

Europanic: 4192

That's a five time difference in murder rate. Rape statistics are even further skewed by counting Hispanics as Europanic, but lets look at that as well.

Black: 24,895

Europanic: 12,571

So even with the fake skew, it's still TWICE as high a rape rate among blacks than Europanics.

Richard Lynn's seminal work "Race Differences in Psychopathic Personality: An Evolutionary Analysis" goes into exhaustive detail. The final report isn't good. Here is an excerpt:

> Nevertheless, as Charles Murray and the late Richard Herrnstein showed in their book *The Bell Curve*, low IQ cannot entirely explain a black crime rate that is six-and-a-half times the white rate. When blacks and whites are matched for IQ, blacks still commit crimes at two-and-a-half times the white rate. This shows that blacks must have some other characteristic besides low intelligence that explains their high levels of criminality.

> Prof. Herrnstein and Dr. Murray found the same race and IQ relationship for social problems other than crime: unemployment, illegitimacy, poverty, and living on welfare. All of these are more frequent among blacks and are related to low IQ, and low IQ goes some way towards explaining them, but these social problems remain greater among blacks than among whites with the same IQ's. Low intelligence is therefore not the whole explanation.

> Prof. Herrnstein and Dr. Murray did not offer any suggestions as to what the additional factors responsible for the greater prevalence of these social problems among blacks might be. They concluded only that "some ethnic differences are not washed away by controlling for either intelligence or for any other variables that we examined. We leave those remaining differences unexplained and look forward to learning from our colleagues where the explanations lie" (p. 340).

I propose that the variable that explains these differences is that blacks are more psychopathic than whites. Just as racial groups differ in average IQ, they can also differ in average levels of other psychological traits, and racial differences in the tendency towards psychopathic personality would explain virtually all the differences in black and white behavior left unexplained by differences in IQ.

Psychopathic personality is a personality disorder of which the central feature is lack of a moral sense. The condition was first identified in the early Nineteenth Century by the British physician John Pritchard, who proposed the term "moral imbecility" for those deficient in moral sense but of normal intelligence.

The term psychopathic personality was first used in 1915 by the German psychiatrist Emile Kraepelin and has been employed as a diagnostic label throughout the Twentieth Century.
In 1941 the condition was described by Hervey Cleckley in what has become a classic book, *The Mask of Sanity*. He described the condition as general poverty of emotional feelings, **lack of remorse or shame,** superficial charm, pathological lying, egocentricity, a lack of insight, absence of nervousness, an inability to love, impulsive antisocial acts, **failure to learn from experience, reckless behavior under the influence of alcohol, and a lack of long-term goals.**

In 1984 the American Psychiatric Association dropped the term psychopathic personality and replaced it with Antisocial Personality Disorder. This is an expression of the increasing sentimentality of the second half of the twentieth century in which terms that had acquired negative associations were replaced by euphemisms.

There are other examples. Mentally retarded children are now called "slow learners" or even "exceptional children;" aggressive children now have "externalizing behaviors;" prostitutes are "sex workers;" tramps are now "the homeless," as if their houses were destroyed by earthquake; and people on welfare are "clients" of social workers. However, the term psychopathic personality remains useful.

…

There is a difference between blacks and whites—analogous to the difference in intelligence—in psychopathic personality considered as a personality trait. Both psychopathic personality and intelligence are bell curves with different means and distributions among blacks and whites. For intelligence, the mean and distribution are both lower among blacks. For psychopathic personality, the mean and distribution are higher among blacks. The effect of this is that there are more black psychopaths and more psychopathic behavior among blacks.

In this we use race merely as a proxy for statistics rather than indicative of Spiteful Mutants, blacks having the most extreme component of their population being spiteful mutants – that does not make all blacks spiteful mutants. Europanics also have spiteful mutants, the disability babies the welfare pond scum and the feminist ass kissing simp men. But it's probably held at about 30% of the males and 60% of the females. Still horrific. Blacks and Hispanics the numbers are probably double that, near complete devastation of the entire race. Not hopeless, but a lot of culling and evolution has to happen to repair what has crept in from 50 years of welfare-ism. Point being, society says never to speak of such things. If we don't confront the truth how do we help them. With MORE handouts, free college, free degrees even though they can't read, and free make work jobs. It's just not the answer. Do they truly contribute after all that? After a make work affirmative action job? Answer: NO

What of those who say its the WELFARE not the RACE? Europanics use welfare as well and on them, especially single mothers, the effect is equally debilitating. And the offspring produced is generally reckless without regard for selecting a quality mate and dysgenic. But it must be more than this. There are genetic factors which predispose races to sloth and welfare parasitism and you will see it across a wide moral compass – single motherhood, drug addiction, inability to hold a job, inability to be educated.

Reduce welfare by 50% and disability payments as well. End nice beautiful section 8 apartments (ok they are slums some places, but other places it results in welfare-ites getting whole beautiful houses). Poverty should be difficult. The poor should never get the same quality housing as the workers. We need a new concept of poor houses, maybe those japanese airport cubes can be a start. 5' high and 4'x10' for a family of four. Crampt, crowded, but a warm roof over your head. No air conditioning. I grew up without it in Texas. The difficulty of it all should allow survival, but not much more, perhaps with a much stronger push than the lavish life of fake nails, fake hair, and 50" tvs and $2000 cell phones, perhaps then the poor might get off their duffs.

Instead, disability is the new path to free and easy living all paid for by our national debt, we can't even afford it today. Its in this population that we breed the gang bangers, the high school drop outs who become murderers, and "oh he had a promising rap career" but never worked a day in his life. We have to recognize the dysgenic nature of welfare but also that it's never the whole story. There is a genetic component, especially among races which have suffered an exhaustion period.

In the meantime, the one resource our nation desperately needs – hard working hard thinking pioneer spirit can do make it happen types – are being force out of existence. This is mainly due to the divorce rape laws but also high taxes but mainly, it's women and feminism and the deciding a childless marriage-less life is better than one with a family. It's going to take some time to start to turn the tide on that, but the divorce rape laws act as rafters propping up that madness and keeping men away. Sure they raped the men and took their piggy banks for 50 years, but now, the words out. It's only the simps and beta cucks who are fair targets anymore, hence a 1.6 replacement rate. We can't move forward when half our population has left the reservation.

The Rise of the Spiteful Mutant population has a direct influence on politics pushing us more and more into Hugo Chavez commie-ism. More poor screaming for more handouts. Twice we have bailed out the bankers. The next bailout might be for the unlanded misery class. Can our monetary system survive another 10T packed on? Probably not but they will do it anyways. We have learned there is no progress to be made neither by DemoThug or RE-blood-ican. Until there is a third party representing Americans, there will be no progress.

Our nation is screaming downhill to a terrifying destiny. Just like so many others that have embraced universal suffrage and las feministas and massive welfare parasitism. Still it's a good watch if only to take not that in the long game China and Europe are more screwed than we are.

The Colluders – Plutocrats, MegaMillionaires, and the FED. Why you are going to be slammed and most big corporations are f-ed

There's some scary stuff going on with bonds and junk ETFs. Most people aren't as familiar with this so I will dive in a bit on what's happened in the simplest terms possible.

Simply stated, dollars are getting vacuumed up and trapped in non-productive caverns. What how eh?

Yes. that's right. Let's take a corporation like Boeing. Let's ride through the full example. This isn't exactly Boeing but you'll get the picture. So there are good times. Companies are profitable. If you look at the example of Carnegie, they use the profits to expand and solidify their business, and put some into savings, which becomes capital for loans and that helps other companies via bank lending. But that's not the new normal in the USA. The new paradigm is one of pure sloth and gluttony. Greed. Most all of the seven deadly sins.

So Boeing, you have to realize ALL the executives all the management team make the big money when the stock price goes up. So doing that in the short term is Job #1. To do this they buy back their stock with their working capital. Often they issue junk debt to fund the stock buybacks which is even worse. Stock prices rise, executives pocket many millions or billions, and they all go off and laugh and buy gold plated yachts. God yacht is hard to spell isnt it?

Now that's all fun and roses until the downturn hits. Now they have all these huge junk bonds. They have no money saved for a rainy day, no if they ever need money they just issue more junk bonds.

Now the FED jumps in. The bonds, especially true horrors like CDOs and other financial scams, get vacuumed up. 3 trillion. 4 trillion. Once the FED starts vacuuming, and they must, because the bonds are worthless and full of grift and crime and that would be made visible if they didn't black hole them. Well, it ain't pretty.

All of this is money. And it all now sits on the FED balance sheet, in debt instruments that sit, or in billionaire's pockets where it mostly sits. None of it makes it to circulate in the regular economy. To see this, pull up "FRED Velocity of Money" and you will see it's a 20 year death spiral straight down. It's not Obama or Trump. Or the virus. Certainly the virus has made things worse. As money is withdrawn from the main street economy and flows only in grifty deals in wall street economy you get a separation of wealth. All the wealth and productivity gains never makes it back to main street. So the working people stagnate and rot.

In the meantime, the politicos get most of their funding from the profits of this grizzy. So will they ever go against it? Not really. Why would they. So we are stuck in this cycle.

The zero to low interest rates make this kind of huxterism easier and seemingly painless as when corporations issue bonds or get loans to do stock buybacks, they do it at a very low interest rate. But in times of crisis, they have used up all their reserves and can't weather a downturn. Boeing now faces only 10% of its seats filled because of the virus. A strong healthy company would weather this. But Boeing needs a bailout to make it. Really the bailout is going straight into the executives pockets, only they stole the money five years ago. So no one can connect the dots.

In response to the vacuum cleaner of the FED, the companies issue completely junk debt to supply the FED and even more profits are made.

Now let's look at the endgame. The FED sits on 3 trillion in buybacks from the 2008 crisis and now has another 4 trillion in buybacks of these dirty financial instruments. They act like they prop up its "balance sheet" but the reality is that they are empty instruments worth nothing. In reality it is NOT an offset of the huge debt. the 28 trillion doesn't get a minus 7 trillion because of the balance sheet of the FED. But they act like it does.

The result – money velocity goes to zero. That's a great depression. And there's no way the fed can get money to main street. Wall street has sealed them in and banks have stopped lending. Just park their money at the fed and get free interest from money they borrowed from the fed for nothing. Or they make real estate loans. All of this is WHY the SBA loan program and the PPP funding is at least in the right direction. But the serfs on main street get loans and interest payments. The plutocrats and executives get free money. free dollars. It's an inherently unfair system.

What happens is you get huge debt burdens on main streets and company failures and closings. Wall street continues to vacuum up dollars and put it in their pockets along with the fat cat executives. Everyone wins but you.

Destroying the Intelligent Class: The H-1B Genocide Visa

One thing that the commies love is to utterly demoralize you. Break your spirit. And then laugh at you. This is the H-1B genocide visa.

For those not in the know, it's a visa for foreign workers, a "non-immigrant" visa but that would be a sham to call it that, but its a sham so ….

It's the non-immigrant visa with which over 40% apply for green cards, get them, and never leave.

It's the visa to bring in third world low IQ savages with fake degrees and fake resumes? What? What do I have to back that up? THREE GAO studies found rampant cheating and fake credentials. THREE.

How many come here? 250-600,000 a year. In recent years the number hovers around 350,000 a year. How many are here? Well if you include those who never left, it's over 4 million. Probably closer to five million.

What lies does the mainstream media say? Well they will declare it's only 85,000 people a year. not true. They will also say it's just a tiny number of the best and brightest. Also not true. Having worked on over 20 projects with teams of these people, they are generally dumb as a stump, stinky, and annoying with their gibberish english. They certainly are not anywhere near the best American engineers.

Why is it a "genocide" visa? Because it's 100% replacement of American engineers. There are only 4 million tech jobs in America and we have over 5 million of these slag labor.

The whole process is rampant with cheating. The placement companies run by Indians are utterly racist and only hire Indians.

Once a curry "nest" is set up, often at prestigious companies like Intel or Oracle, all they hire are more Indians. If an American does end up in a curry den, they don't last long. Either they get tasked to fix the mess the Indians and Chinese created, or it's just a grim place to be with stupidity running rampant.

It gets worse. They go to congress and claim they can't find Americans to hire (LIE) and then bring in tens of thousands of foreign fake engineers, finally they layoff their best and brightest.

Now, a company can't lay off their best and brightest engineers that wouldn't be in their own interest you say. Well, you see all the upper management is WHITE in these companies. So they NEED the brown staff to make it seem like they are "diverse" all of this is an exercise in diversity and also, it's a denigration of the engineering class. The MBAs despise engineers because engineers are much much smarter than MBAs. But the MBAs can layoff whole swaths of Americans and pocket a tidy bonus for "saving money" with the cheaper H-1B workers.

You will notice this only happens in mature successful companies. They can rape it like this for about 10 years before they start to get major failures that can't be hidden. Boeing's engine design disaster didn't happen until they let go a whole team of senior engineers. And they have a UNION!

Project after project results in failure. The H-1B workers often just pretend to work or do total fraud jobs. I've caught them personally in major fraud at five major fortune 100 companies and on over ten contracts. What kind of fakery? Pretending tests are real, pretending the code is working, or just covering for each other when only 1 out of the 20 engineers can actually produce anything at all. The others are just seat warmers. The company thinks they are saving money over an expensive American engineer but the truth is they are paying 10 times more.

I can't prove it, but I think there's one other thing going on. Companies essentially have these workers as slaves. They so hope to get green card sponsorship to get out of shit hole china and india that they put up with all kinds of abuse – long hours, being treated like shit, etc. It's a superiority complex for the slime MBAs.

This has happened to IBM, Oracle, Disney, Intel, Microsoft. It's EVERYWHERE. It's now so endemic that if they canceled the H-1B visa today Americans would STILL never get jobs.

This is demoralizing our best and brightest. It's outrageous, it's well known, and no politician will do anything about it. The big silicon valley campaign handouts are at risk.

Even when American engineers have jobs, they have suffered terrible salary stagnation vs. what they would be earning if this genocide had not taken place.

No one cares because America as a nation doesn't give shit. One more sign of the collapse to a land of spiteful mutants. It's pathetic.

The Great Trump Failure and "Undocumented Neighbors"

I'm watching Tucker Carlson and he has on some hispanic who keep referring to illegal alien invader criminals as "undocumented neighbors". I don't have words.

Trump really wrecked the nation forever by breaking all his promises. Why does this keep happening. There wont be even a hope of salvation or change no matter what they promise unless it comes from a new third party. That's what we have learned. Unfortunately, it's already too late, the damage done, we are hopelessly FKED at this point.

First promise broke – End Birthright citizenship. This is perhaps the most damaging of all. There is no LAW that says if you are born here you become a citizen. Even Tucker fell for it spouting that the "neighbors" guy was a citizen. No he's not. There is no such thing as birthright citizenship for invaders. This means that the 100 million illegal alien invaders currently here in our country have children who seem to be "defacto" recognized as citizens, even given social security numbers! MADNESS. Oh but the Trump Fk-ing goes on and on.

Second promise broke – to END the H-1B genocide visa. Thats where they take our best and brightest engineers, kick them in the teeth and throw them into the streets and replace them with Sanjay and his fake degree from India. 5 million of them now. There are only 4 million computer jobs in America.

Third promise broke – Lock her up. She's still free last I checked. And what happened to prosecuting the criminals in the CIA and FBI. Durhams report never comes. Trey gowdy just announced "don't expect prosecutions". They cover for their own.

What mistake did Trump make? He brought in the WORST DC insiders to run everything, and they damn well like what's going on.

DACAns – the illegal children who snuck into America? He could Thanos snap them away. Sanctuary cities? He could arrest those mayors and put them in the hoose gaw where they belong.

The Demothugs, being the pure evil party hell bent on the total destruction of the nation to stay in power, make voting Republoblood seem like a good choice. It isn't.

Now we have an insidious plot to fake count corona virus deaths. Keep the shutdown going even if it means collapsing the economy to great depression levels. The CDC issued a notice that we could count "suspected" cases as deaths. with no proof. And the cheating began there. It's going to be damn obvious soon when America's curve doesn't follow any other nations.

The FED acted again to take CDOs and CMOs into their wing stuffed with failed loans and fraudulent double booked mortgages. The bankers and huxsters stuffed billions into their own pockets. This is the second time it's happened, pushing our debt up to 28 trillion. Never again I thought? But apparently no one cares.

This nation is sick of the invaders, sick of throwing our best and brightest into the streets but it's all going forward full bore under trump. "I'll build dah wall" says Trump. I think we got 50 miles last I checked.

So I've changed my mind. I was optimistic I thought that if we delayed we could somehow overcome and change our fate. No longer. America is flat out doomed.

After the Red Pill Rage – Your Relation with Bythus – A Deeper Obscured Sacred that Wittgenstein told us about and Nan Chu'an Did Not

The red pill rage is a stage in the MGTOW grief cycle (men going their own way, opting out of marriage and relationships due to unfair courts, rape charges and divorce rape).

But the red pill rage can occur any time we wake up from THOU SHALT. It occurs when we realize the path we have so dutifully followed is a fraud, a lie, a control. So it's not just mgtow, its a state of spirit.

All too often, this results in despair and suicide. But make it past this and you will be left in a enuii state, lost wandering. In my earlier days I called it dwelling. The goal should be to convert this to sacred dwelling, once past the rat race, the goat pulling the wagon to the point of exhaustion, and once past the rage, there is a pause. a silence.

Once silent, there is a possibility to observe the sacred. But, your muscles for that are far too weak. That is why in Buddhism there is the beginners practice. Just coming to quiet is not enough to observe of the sacred. It takes work, and not the stuff they do in church.

If you do not become aware of the sacred, you will become lost in a logico-analytico mindset which is never fulfilling. You may begin to better understand the enslaving systems, but that won't ever make you feel better. So this next transitive step is very important in dealing with the world, especially a world in crisis, a world where the spiteful mutants are getting all the rewards and you are seen just as a work goat to siphon off wealth to keep a system from hyper-inflating. That's what taxes do. that's why taxes are so high. And that's why bankers keep getting bailouts for faulty loans and CMOs while the serfs get 22% credit card loans. It's designed to keep you on the precipice of failure, helpless and hopeless, WORK HARDER GOAT. And most do.

The red pill rage is not enough to wake up from their spell. It's more like having a first nightterror and waking up screaming. It's not enough to quite understand the dreaming state you have lived your whole life in.

The concept of WAKING UP runs through sacred literature. What does that mean, I'm awake. No, you are still in a dream.

It is Nan Chu'an's peony, a Classic Zen Koan (life teaching story)

"People see this flower as if in a dream" says the teacher.

Not in a dream. But as if in a dream. The enslaved state.

We learn more from Nan Chu'an in a follow up Koan

Nan Ch'uan went to see Master Nirvana of Pai Chang (Mountain.)

Chang asked, "Have all the sages since antiquity had a truth that they haven't spoken for people?"

Ch'uan said, "They have."

Chang said, "What is the truth that hasn't been spoken for people?"

Ch'uan said, "It's not mind, it's not buddha, it's not any thing."

Chang said, "You said it."

Ch'uan said, "I am just thus. What about you, Teacher?"

Chang said, "I am not a great man of knowledge either: how would I know whether it has been spoken or not?"

Ch'uan said, "I don't understand."

Chang said, "I've already spoken too much for you."

Chu'an replies in the most important and sincere way – "I am just thus" this is powerful teaching. He is already far down the path. It is not Mind not Buddha, not anything. Powerful knowledge. It takes drunken old men 100 lifetimes to get to such knowledge.

Chang admonishes him. I've already said too much. Why? Because you have to realize it yourself. **Your freedom is your burden**. Only you can awaken yourself, not words of sages.

> "And becoming aware of one's true inner nature, instinctive gut feelings, is not generally thought by those who experience it to be in conflict with the essence of one's spiritual knowledge, but more of a Gnostic direct experience of the Sacred experienced in the gut or all of nature that is greater than us and is connected to us through the gut instincts."
> — Martha Char Love, What's Behind Your Belly Button? A Psychological Perspective of the Intelligence of Human Nature and Gut Instinct

The main issue is a rejection of the God of the Old Testament as a false god who made a mistake by creating the world. Jesus is held up as a teacher of whatever school of gnosticism was quoting him, and he is always set in opposition to the god of the Old Testament.

Generally, the true god, in their opinion, was unknowable. In fact, often they referred to him as *Bythus*, which means "deep" or "profound."

It is your relationship with Bythus that will fundamentally change your world. We start out as logic creatures. Deep in analyzing and classifying. Deep in thirst for Sophia, our questing for ever more science and knowledge. And we travel that path until we hit the walls of our prison. We then confront THOU SHALT and rage against, a fierce lion, endlessly roaring for our freedom never to come. And then finally, we transform again into a spiritual being, a innocent child, a newness against the universe, because we know the Bythus, and we are still, and finally in that stillness, we can grasp the sacred.

"They maintain that Daniel also set forth the same thing when he begged of the angels explanations of the parables, as being himself ignorant of them. But the angel, hiding from him the great mystery of Bythus, said to him, Go your way quickly, Daniel, for these sayings are closed up until those who have understanding do understand them, and those who are white be made white. Moreover, they boast that they are the *white* and the men of *good understanding*."- Against Heresies, I.19 (St. Irenaeus)

Wittgenstein also taught of what we cannot know about.

Wittgenstein writes, "**Not how the world is the mystical**, but that it is." He elaborates: "We feel that even if all possible scientific questions be answered, the problems of life have still not been touched at all. Of course there is then no question left, and just this is the answer.

"My propositions serve as elucidations in the following way: anyone who understands me eventually recognizes them as nonsensical, when he has used them – as steps – to climb up beyond them. (He must, so to speak, throw away the ladder after he has climbed up it.) He must transcend these propositions, and then he will see the world aright. What we cannot speak about we must pass over in silence"

And in that silence, we become open to the sacred, the mystical, that is, to see the world sub specie aeterni – under the guise of eternity."

Wittgenstein tells us again in his lectures on ethics:

"I now see that these nonsensical expressions were not nonsensical because I had not yet
found the correct expressions, but that their nonsensicality was their very essence. For all I wanted to do with them was just to go beyond the world and that is to say beyond significant language. My whole tendency and I believe the tendency of all men who ever tried to write or talk Ethics or Religion was to run against the boundaries of language. This running against the walls of our cage is perfectly, absolutely hopeless."

Knowing our walls our cage is the first step to overcoming them. Coming at rest in our cage is the first step to being open to the sacred.

"(6.44) It is not *how* things are in the world that is mystical, but *that* it exists. (6.45) To view the world sub specie aeterni is to view it as a whole – a limited whole. (6.45) Feeling the world as a limited whole – it is this that is mystical. When the answer cannot be put into words, neither can the question be put into words. The *riddle* does not exist. […] (6.522)" – TLP

In Buddhism they talk of the one and the ten thousand things. You being is a place that a river of eternity runs through. Do you look back at the river exiting you or forward to the eternity approaching you? Where do you find you. Where do you find world. In the instant, open to the sacred, beyond words, you see it with direct pointing to the true nature of reality. You find it by first becoming a still vessel, turbulent water does not reflect the moon.

It is something most never see, most never glipse or obtain. Sammadhi, a mere instant glimpse into the true reality, is enough to cause us to change our whole lifetimes.

It is this attainment that Marcus' disciples try to discuss...

"[Marcus' disciples] maintain that they have attained to a height above all power and that therefore they are free in every respect to act as they please, having no one to fear in anything."

True freedom. We saw the same in the Buddha, in the early Christians. Free from the rules of the grown society that entrapped us for so long.

"For they say that because of the redemption they can now neither be stopped nor even seen by the judge. And even if he should happen to lay hold on them, then they can simply repeat these words ... : "O you who sit beside God and the mystical, eternal Sige [*Silence*]," – (Against Heresies I:13:6)

They direct judges that they cannot judge with words. And that is correct.

"you through whom the angels—who continually behold the face of the Father and have you as their guide and introducer—derive their forms from above ... Behold, the judge is at hand, and the crier orders me to make my defense. But I ask you, as being acquainted with the affairs of both, to present the cause of both of us to the judge, inasmuch as it is in reality but one cause." – (Against Heresies I:13:6)

In a land of all one, from one source, there can be no other, no judges.

"Now, as soon as the Mother hears these words, she puts the Homeric helmet of Pluto [*which makes men invisible*] upon them so that they may invisibly escape the judge." – (Against Heresies I:13:6)

The free men get the gift of this invisibility.

"Every one of them generates something new, day by day, according to his ability, for no one is deemed "perfect," who does not develop among them some mighty fictions. : -(Against Heresies I:18:1)

And that is the powerful lesson. Freed of the constraints, knowing the scacred, one creates something new every day. The point of your existence. Laid bare. Such is the woe of the non-creators, the cube bound, the on disability coffee house dwellers and all forms of Spiteful Mutants, the on disability adult babies, the fem-men in pink, the teachers who teach nothing and create nothing, the derelicts and morphine addicts who see only the cage and never the freedom. Knowing them, you chose to never become them nor never bound by them or their false teachings nor that of the chains of society – the rules of marriage, divorce, and the lack of free movement and free land. The restriction of all freedoms, more chains. I seek a better place where I can be free. That is my driving force.

The Debt, Higher Taxes, Inflation, Poorer Middle Class, Fewer Children Cycle

Ah DEBT. It must be DEBT that is stopping Americans from having babies ... or is it insane divorce courts raping our men'? Whites have stopped having children altogether. Fear not, they do not include the 10 million who sneak into our country every year illegally.

It's a vicious cycle. That pizza I could get for a cheap $2.50 meal is now $4.00. That's a price that's nearly doubled in just ten years. On average, if you consider more real measures of inflation (see shadowstats) our currency is losing at least 50% of its value every decade. The dumb pidgeon middle class sees 401k accounts and their home values going up and thinks it's a good thing. No it's part of a lethal cycle. It ends in more poverty and fewer productive people able to have children. Its those on welfare who have the security to make babies not our best and brightest.

Career salaries have also changed dramatically over the past 20 years. Doctors, Lawyers, and Engineers used to make about the same. Now doctors and big business lawyers routinely earn over $400,000 a year. They are hedged against inflation. Doctors through government payola and insurance companies which hide fees that would normally make us vomit if paid directly. Lawyers do better as they are parasites off the Fatcat corporations which feed on us. College bureaucrats used to make a trifling, now 800,000 salaries aren't uncommon. Janet Reno got over a million a year.

But more and more, as our investments yield turn to 1 or 2% retirement accounts for municipalities which give all their workers and firemen and police fat retirement packages need to claw the money to pay for that largess from somewhere.

So they hit the middle class with ridiculous unaffordable property taxes, often more than 600 a month for modest homes in modest states.

All of this has the effect to burn out the middle class. it's a tired people more and more feeling forgotten. Trumps rev to the economy just began to lift people up when the virus struck.

Looking at the annual US population growth, the deceleration from 1790 to present isn't hard to see, but the sharp collapse in growth due to influenza at the end of WWI takes a little closer look. However, after the influenza was contained by 1920'ish, the under 65 year-old growth rate immediately recovered to trend growth before continuing its deceleration.

It just so happens that 2019 and 1918/1919 had something very important in common, they were the only years in US history with population decline among the under 65 year-old population. As per the Census, (HERE), while the total US population grew by 1.55 million (0.48%) in 2019, all the net population growth came among the 65+ year-old population (which grew about 1.625 million). This means that in 2019, the under 65 year-old population declined by about 70 thousand. The only time this ever occurred previously in US history was at the height of a global pandemic. Yet, there was no pandemic in 2019...just a population unwilling to enter into parenthood at record proportions and immigration rates about half of what they were during the previous decade. Of course, if a pandemic were to hit now with an under 65 year-old annual growth rate already below anything the US has ever experienced, the population declines would naturally be unlike anything the US has ever seen.

The rationale for the continued declining fertility rates and births appears to be the continued growth of federal debt well in advance of economic activity. The mounting $23+ trillion in federal debt (and quadruple that in unfunded liabilities) will never be repaid and can't honestly be serviced at anything but Federal

Reserve dictated minimal interest rates.

Thus, the Fed continues to rig the interest rates, which rigs stocks and commodities…and the outcome is unnaturally high asset appreciation…which rewards elderly and institutional asset holders and punishes young, poor, and those absent assets. Young and poor are suffering from costs of living rising far faster than incomes.

Marriage are being put off and the undertaking of childrearing is a choice that can simply be avoided with widely available birth control. Simply put, it is the Federal Reserve coping mechanisms that are causing record low fertility rates as young adults are financially unable/unwilling to undertake children. The Fed is preserving the present for the elderly and institutions at the expense of the young and poor present and future.

Absolutist Right – Dysgenics vs. Welfare, and Race — Which is the underlying principle affecting society?

One of the mistakes people make in looking at the genetic basis of IQ, behaviour, and psychopathology (violence) is they will cite a case where in one group they have a higher IQ but also higher psychopathology. But this is poor genetics. If you consider that races have different clusters of these factors. They are not cross-linked to the same gene. So they can exist in variety. So we might have a group like Native Americans, who have slightly higher IQ than Hispanics but much higher psychopathology. Or you might consider American blacks, who have europanic admixture in their genetics. They are higher IQ than african blacks (15 points) but still suffer from much higher rates of psychopathology.

So one argument goes, well it's all genetic. If you put one race of people on an island, fast forward 300 years, they will probably end up looking much like their source nation. Liberia or Haiti are historical examples. We also have the mostly post Caucasian South Africa. South Africa and other AFrican nations – Zimbabwe, Congo – that threw out Europanics – given 100 years will descend pretty much back to the state when the Explorers found them. Sewage systems break and never get fixed. In Guatemala in Antigua they have the collapsed spanish churches that the natives have no understanding how to fix.

If you accept this genetic fatalism, then the changing racial profile of America alarms you. Its doom. The end. And the immigrant invasion or breeding of dysgenics is not simply troublesome its a full on existential crisis.

There is evidence that supports this. There have been several twin studies where one was raised in a more affluent area, and in this case a black youth ended up still violent and disruptive and failed to learn much, regardless of the higher income level. Really the higher income merely shields these traits and makes them harder to see, but they are still there. So Affirmative action is not only wrong, its a wasted effort.

"We conclude that there is now strong evidence that virtually all individual psychological differences, when reliably measured, are moderately to substantially heritable." – Genetic and environmental influences on human psychological differences, Journal of Neurobiology 54(1):4-45 · January 2003

Similary its a grab bag, being high IQ does not necessarily mean you are getting all positive genes:

> Ashkenazi Jews are 40% more likely than ethnic Europeans to carry genes associated with schizophrenia and with bipolar disorder [Genome-wide association study of schizophrenia in Ashkenazi Jews, by F. Goes et al., *American Journal of Medical Genetics,* 2015]. Schizophrenia makes you paranoid about people and causes you see evidence agency and conspiracies everywhere. Bipolar disorder causes you to perceive the world in a very negative way and fixate on the worst possible outcome.

In his new book, *Blueprint: How DNA Makes Us Who We Are*, Plomin takes recent genetic research and draws some provocative conclusions

Plomin believes that Freud sent society looking in the wrong place for answers to the question of what makes us as we are. The key to personality traits does not lie in how you were treated by your parents, but rather in what you inherited biologically from them: namely, the genes in your DNA.

He finds that genetic heritability accounts for 50% of the psychological differences between us, from personality to mental abilities. But that leaves 50% that should be accounted for by the environment. However, Plomin argues, research shows that most of *that* 50% is not attributable to the type of environmental influences that can be planned for or readily affected.

And this is where epi-genetics comes into play. In countries which had severely malnourished children, IQs will rise given the right diet and supplements. But never above their genetic threshold.

Similarly, blacks, who are higher in psychopathology than any other race, given strong parental structure and well organized controlled education, they too will rise, but only to the peak of their genetic threshold. This will be well above the mean, but probably only low-average compared to Europanics.

Does this mean it's a doom sentence to be born into a dysgenic race? Hardly. There are so many traits which some races will excel. Jazz music for example is chock full of black pioneers in music. Rocket scientists? Not so much (and no – hidden figures is a myth, read our article on that non-sense here).

However, when planning for populations, you cannot consider the outliers and begin to look at things from a mean. We know that city by city, once they become more than 50% Non-Europanic (unless it has a large asian component) it descends into poverty and violence just like the races exhibit globally.

Asians are a somewhat complex race group and also not always a positive. They tend to be conforming and non-inventive. Smarter than average Europanics perhaps only because so many Europanics are coddled and don't study. Which would be unthinkable in most Asian households. Studying and solving problems is another way to extend the genetic threshold of IQ, literally strengthening and growing connections in the brain. If you don't do it, you end up dumb as a rock.

However, that doesn't mean that a city that was 100% asian would be ideal either. Sure it may be low crime, but it would probably stagnate and cease having babies our of sheer boredom and introvertedness.

So an ideal society is probably a bit more Brave New World than Master Race. You do need the laborers, factory workers, social workers, garbage men, as well as the inventors and entrepreneurs and even the slimy financial class to get it all working. Am I build to plow the fields? Probably not.

But Dysgenics means you have affronted natural selection. Take eye glasses. No longer are people with poor vision weeded out, so we are dependent on glasses. With welfare, no longer are those who can't earn enough to feed themselves weeded out. Dysgenics effects many many traits and only in competition will it end.

After a war when you lose and are mostly wiped out of your best men (post WWII Germany) you will see the rise of ... for better words ... "girly-men" and weak peoples and eventually Angela Merkel is the best leader they can produce. This is dysgenics. Slavery also had a large dysgenic effect on blacks, as the rebellious and strong were weeded out, and the more simpleton were kept to work the fields. This may explain why Africans who come from Africa to the USA exhibit strong entrepreneurship while many native Blacks seem more like children needing parents. But we can't say that because that's RACIST (aka we understand racial differences. Who isn't racist except a dimwitted fool?)

What of the argument that it's welfare and feminism that has wrecked society and certain groups. The answer is tha's true as well. Welfare has ruined our society especially women who now marry the government. Choosing a good mate is no longer required, they can party through their 30s and not worry. That's the dysgenic effect of welfare that most don't think of.

So these are not either or beliefs. They are both multi-factorial contributing factors to the destruction of our society. Which is more important is debatable, but it doesn't change the fact that we need to make progress on both fronts. Sadly we are doing all of this at breakneck speed hurtling to our doom. what to take on first? We have to take on all if it. Or just leave and watch the starving multitudes eat each other from afar.

Section 8 housing is particularly deplorable. There should be a lower standard of housing for the poor. In England, its much worse, muslim families of 12 get full on victorian mansions to live in. We aren't quite that stupid in the USA. But nearly.

Why fight at all if we are doomed? One answer is Sweden and France. The hope is that if we SEE these nations collapse in 15 years there might be time to hard brake and make the big changes. It's a hopeful thought, better than knowing the money runs out in 2035. Italy with its no babies is also growing old and dying off.

Ultimately reducing welfare and making it truly miserable, with punishments not rewards for having children, and rewards for not having children (the 180 from what we do now), changing the class of housing you get, and suddenly being a welfare momma with 12 chillin isn't as good looking a deal.

Education reform where we can allow our gifted children to go at full pace and not be held back to the dumb mean or distruptive classrooms will also be a big leap forward and there's no reason to not do this.

Divorce reform and ending the raping of men would let men back into the marriage market.

And finally genetic reform, the most controversial, where we try to return to a historical productive america which was 90% Europanic, should be a basis for our policies as a nation. If we are replaced by people from Haiti, then we will become Haiti. If we are replaced by people from the middle east or Africa, we will end up looking like those places.

There are no easy answers. Probably the shifts required will never happen. Things will get worse and worse. Our only salvation is that other nations are ahead of us in their collapse. We might wake up. But change wouldn't happen without a third political party in America, the two we have now don't care about these issues whatsoever, regardless of broken Trump campaign platitudes.

The Extinction Party – The New Democrats and the End of America

The democrats have pivoted to pure Marxist – underclass – victimhood – racial division as their mantra. And we know that philosophy well:

The Jews – Israel – 22 Million Dead

The Jews – Stalin – Ukraine and Russia – 80 Million Dead

Mao – China – 100 Million Dead

And our current examples of Venezuela.

America has acted to push a light form of socialism, but it's getting worse. More and more money for handouts, scammers double dipping, working under the table, getting grants as care givers and babysitters. Welfare wasn't meant to be a get rich scheme, but it's funding upper middle class lives through abuse and graft. And the people it has produced is the insane GIBSMEDAT culture. And another 50 million in caravans knocking on our fences trying to push them over to get on the gravy train.

For sure, we aren't as horrific as England – giving multimillion dollar houses to Middle Eastern and Indian families with 12 children. For free. We aren't as insane as Germany, welcoming in 2 million black muslim invaders and giving them free housing, money, computers, video games, and then with all their leisure time they go out and rape 8 year old girls.

We aren't yet as horrific as Sweden, where the pink waisted cucked males nod as bitchy female leaders talk about the need to suck the Negros balls and have their babies.

Well. What are we going to do. We have let in so MANY dysgenic people who are on the government dole one way or another, or simply own real estate that all these invaders prop the price up on, that the entire Democratic opposition party has changed from a pro Worker advocate to a DESTROY AMERICA DESTROY THE WORKERS fang toothed insanity party.

I call them the extinction party. Because IF we ever do follow their plans it will result in the extinction of our people – the free-est, brightest, most industriest peoples ever to form a nation. And that is a forever card, a truly shocking future that I cannot help but fight against.

All of the Democrat agenda seems like a horrific Communist plot to destroy the nation.

They push for endless immigration, ending our borders, even ending all border ICE enforcement agents. They push sanctuary cities. They push for voter fraud – no ID and mail in ballots. Worse ballot dumping, literally you are legally able to drop of a truck of filled in ballots. Then when Trump tried to investigate for voter fraud in California – Nah uh – they wouldn't let him in.

The pushing for endless minority rights and free handouts – free college free healthcare free welfare free dollars. Bernie Sanders "socialism" is just a proxy for communism. Which always leads to despotic dictatorship. The slaughter of Ukraine should give you pause.

The democratic party used to be for the workers. Now it's just a full on push for authoritarian control in some warped communist-dictatorship. Domme-unist party. They are ANTI-America. They are the party of the spiteful mutants. The lower heard non producers. They hear and represent THAT voice. So it's literally the producers against the non-producers EXCEPT the Re-Bloodicans haven't stood up to them in any way. They are spineless and useless. So the productive working class and middle class Americans have no political representation. We thought it was Trump but he lied. There won't be any representation until there is a third political party. But the flood of immigrants and welfare thuggies will increase faster than that can be formed. It's literally a race. Will we get there and block the floodgates before we drown? Maybe not. Trump may be the last republican president. It may swing all democratic forever after that. Once Texas falls that's all they need to rule forever. That's the democratic game plan. Win by destroying the nation. It should unsettle everyone, but the spiteful mutants don't care. Gibs-me-dat and the world's unfair and racist clouds their mind like a Sith paduwan. They are like hungry pigs eating their slop mindlessly. And they are our doom.

For them it's a win. Free education, free welfare/disability, free housing, hubby works under the table for cash, and they basically have a upper middle class lifestyle including healthcare, something a lot of the middle class can't afford. As the handouts become OBVIOUSLY better than trying to work for a living, people will just go "fk it" and run to the dark side. It's already happening.

Rise of the Dark State

People are often confused about Fascism. Let's start with Communism. Communism is a one party system that can never lose power in elections. Communism promotes shared not private property, and in its worst form dictates the type of labor one must perform (sending professors to grow rice).

Fascism is also a one party system that remains in power. But it still has and respects private property and the rights of business. The problem with Fascism is the only government examples – WWII era Germany and Italy – were stuck in a war cycle. We really cannot know the non-war cycle fascism. Does Fascism lead inexorably to war? We can't know that. It certainly by definition doesn't require it. The unification of ones split off peoples was a standard effort of WWII resulting from artificial country boundaries drawn at the end of WWI.

So now what do we have in the united states. Well we have a two party system but there can never be a strong 3rd party the way the system is designed. And on many points the two parties do not differ as much as one would think. So it's not quite one party, but its not much more than one party either. It's an illusion of choice to fool the people.

And what about private property in America? There is none. They tax property at huge insane rates that means you never can feel secure or really own your property. Interestingly, Neither Hitler Nor China had such property taxes. China still doesn't! Which is why housing speculation is rampant.

Some say Hitler took the guns. Alex Jones comes to mind. But he didn't. He believed in an armed citizenry like Switzerland.

The point is, thinking that America is somehow a saintly system better than Fascism is incorrect. We only understand Hitler's fascist Germany from a war footing. We don't understand nor can we predict what it could have become. But if we look at the pre-war accomplishments of Fascism it was dramatic. Starving people were fed, highways were built, economy was restored, people were happy again and things were booming. And Jews were gassed and pushed into ovens you say. Well, maybe, maybe not. There's not much proof for that. Worse, International Jews had declared an import ban on German Goods which would have starved Germany. Jews were seen as non-germans for good reason. The plan was to re-settle them, but the jewish leaders opposed settlement anywhere but Palestein which of course Germany had no legal jurisdiction over. So things bogged down with many Jews using the offer for resettlement in Spain.

Fascism. Hitler. Evil. Really when I look at the USA I think much of what we think is free and fair elections are now mostly faked. Ballot dumping was just made illegal. Democrats have been caught time and time again stuffing the ballot boxes with illegals who should never have been on the voting roles, they oppose voter ID and worse they refused the investigation into the 2016 votes and refused to turn over anything. What do they have to hide? Oh not much, just that they have been faking elections everywhere they get into power.

The democrats are the new communists willing to cheat and do whatever it takes to seize power and then, as a communist system will ensure they never ever lose power. this has happened to California and New York. Now they are trying (and thank goodness failing) to turn Texas commie red.

So Trumps effort to restrain illegal immigration is in effect against the commie takeover of our nation. Only idiots will be for that. Sadly, the feminine need for protectionism has led many native people into wishing for a communist police state without knowing it. And they see the embracing of all foreign peoples as motherly love for strangers. But these aren't our tribe, they aren't our people. This is Violent Altruisn gone amok and it will be the end of us. Subverting the masculine is directly involved in this effort.

When I look at the mess America is in, Fascism seems a lot better. Private Property, Free and Productive industry, and strong Christian values. In the end, we might have to turn to a Fascist system to block out the communists. That would be a sad day, but preferential over the mass genocide and starvation that always follows communism. Fascism seems Patriarchial. Communism Matriarchal. Two systems in violent opposition.

All of the efforts of communists to take hold have been through arguing a false straw man placed in front of them to hide their true nature. Anti-Masculinity. Climate Change. Pro-LGBT. Pro-Negroid. Pro-Invasion. All of these efforts are simply masks over the evils of communism. Because our society has been filled with unproductive dysgenic races, dysgenic peoples, who cannot win in fair capitalism and instead want the government to give them the upper hand. This has already happened with women being granted no-fault divorce, cushy Alimony, and enough freebies that marriage just isn't palatable to them anymore. Sure they are emancipated, to nowhere childless and alone. It's a system that does not produce children and in 20 years the population exhaustion will cause the welfare state to blow up. Will the taxes from the newly dysgenic peoples of the US who already need disability checks for thuh 'chillin support the elderly retirees? Nope.

We are in a death endgame. Against the communists. And for them, villifying fascism and cowering behind democracy (which our founders never supported, we are a republic not a democracy) already they have corrupted congress by having all the illegals counted giving them too many seats in congress. And when Trump tried to get the citizenship question on the census and they pushed back he cucked out like a castrated harem guard. When will we ever get someone with the balls to change this obviouos corrupted farce the demothugs have been playing for 20 years now?

How Welfare and Parasitism from Blacks and Invaders Impoverishes the Middle Class via Exorbitant Property Taxes

The cost for the dysgenic transformation of the U.S.A from a Europanic nation with 9% non-europanics to a hodge podge society with 50% non-Europanics is shuttered upon the middle class in the form of property taxes.

Property taxes essentially turn America into a communist nation. There is no private property, everything is a loan from the state. That is exactly how they do it in China.

And rising property taxes are now required to support the huge pensions for the dumb people – the teachers, the police officers, the government workers, etc – while the smart hard working people generally are told "get a 401k" ha ha ha suckers.

The extreme welfare parasitism – ghetto mommas with ten chillin getting $2000 a month and a free house – and the refugee industry funnelling billions to the "charities" for housing and resettlement, and then the welfare comes. It's all adding to the massive taxes on the middle class. The Trump tax break? It didn't lower taxes. We lost the deduction for interest on mortgage and rates actually increased for the upper middle class, in exchange for a higher standard deduction. For most of the middle class it was a wash. the real benefits were of course given to the corporations.

But the low interest rates, which were caused from overspending on warfare and welfare which forces america to run at a 1 trillion dollar deficit each year – requires the low interest rates or America would be instantly bankrupt. But those same low interest rates make the 7% projected returns on the pension funds nearly impossible. Which is why the FED and FOMC pressured the largest corporations to use the corporate tax break to buy back stocks raising the markets and fluffing pension funds.

But at the municipal level, these pension costs leave them no recourse except to drive up property taxes. To a ridiculous level. And this is the doom of the middle class.

It's a complex dance. Many steps in between. So most people cannot understand that it is our move to a dysgenic welfare nation and prison nation of the poor genetics and high psychopathy races that all are a net drain on society, basically they overwhelm the Europanics production. 40% dysgenic was the tipping point and now we are at 50% dysgenic and running headlong into 70% dysgenic population by 2050. This is a doomsday scenario but much too complex for the regular American to follow.

Multi-culturalism, invasion, our welfare state, all must be changed. So what to do?

FIRST, end birthright citizenship recognition. It was never legally recognized and should not be the law. Trump can change this with a EO and a bureaucratic change.

SECOND, end ALL payola and welfare for invaders, illegals, and refugees UNTIL they obtain their green cards.

THIRD, change the welfare system so that there is a FIXED RATE regardless of the number of children AND a bonus to women for not having any children.

That is not enough to save us, but it will slow down the ghetto-ization of America. And maybe as we watch Sweden fail and burn to the ground we might just wake up and restore our Europanic nation.

An even more equitable solution would be to end welfare altogether, and every American who earns under $200k would have the option to request $1000 a month. Many wouldn't take the money. But, and this is where the Yang Gang FAILS, is that you must then end all welfare, section 8, food stamps, money for "chillin" AND on top of that you have to stop giving disability for having an IQ which is representative of your race. We cannot give out disability payola if you are negro and have a 80 IQ because that is normal. Also, disability payola must be based on a working income for the average of the past 10 years. If you haven't put in 10 years, no disability. That would stop asians importing their grandmothers and mothers and immediately putting them on disability roles.

And of course, if you aren't a citizen you get NADA. Green card holder? NADA. And of course that leads us to BirthRight citizenship reform, which NEVER existed as a law and NO the 14th amendment doesn't confer it. You must have ONE PARENT who is an American Citizen to confer citizenship on the child.

All of this has to happen all together. And much of it can be done via executive order as much of this is administrative and reflects the payola back to the states for welfare. If a state like CAli wants to bankrupt itself by handing out welfare payments to illegal invaders, so be it, but no more Obama bailouts to California like we have done in the past.

Psychopathology and Race

We need to recognize that Europanics and Africans diverged over a MILLION YEARS ago, our difference is NOT skin deep. Not only in intelligence, but also in PsychoPathology (proclivity towards murder, rape, theft, and rampaging looting and burning) is clearly different among the races as well.

When someone tells you you are a "Racist" say yes my brain functions well I can recognize and clearly detail the differences in the races of Man, when they diverged, their differences in IQ and Psychopathology. **What is my ERROR. WHAT IS MY ERROR?** And are you not RETARDED for not being able to do so?

Also, when they tell you we must take in Refugees from War Torn Africa, say Why? War is what African peoples do. They are in their natural state. Surely we do not want their violence and anger here.

Also, when they tell you we must take in Refugees because of drought tell them, wait a second, is there a drought, or did they fail to plan, breed endlessly, and destroy their habitat. We don't want those inferior genetic traits here!

Blacks clearly have hugely elevated testosterone much earlier than Europanics, by the mid 30s Europanics catch up as African testosterone dwindles. This is one reason why the African children teens and early adults are such handfuls and difficult to educate, and post a fake schooling become unable to fit into the work-a-day culture of Europanics. Just as bodybuilders who take steroids are prone to anger and fighting, the same is the case with Black males except for them it's simply genetics, no doubt a POSITIVE trait for survival in Afrika, and a horrible trait for fitting in modern society. Interestingly enough, the college bound tend to have much lower levels of T for both Europanics and Blacks.

Now, our education system could compensate for this difference if it were allowed to recognize it (its not) and vary the education given to blacks. This has already defacto happened in inner city schools except, they threw all education away and are basically baby sitters. With on-line education and evaluation there is zero need for this. Let people learn at their own pace, take breaks to let off steam, and then return to learning. But the teachers unions cannot stop feeling their own self aggrandizement for teaching them little more than to tie their shoes.

Europanics similarly could get a education that stressed their invention and high IQ, and asians would fall somewhere in the middle. But thats RACIST. Everyone is the same. So we produce armies that cannot read upon high school graduation.

First principle, recognizing and understanding these differences is pivotal to correcting the failure of American education.

Are east asians outdistancing Europanics on IQ? Well it's not as clear cut as the chart shows. Europanics still have a lot of dumb people to weed out, and sadly our welfare programs help them to outbreed the rest of us. That's dysgenics. But there is another side which is the creative / inventive side which IQ tests do not measure at all. And on this front, the Europanics are far out front which is the main reason why China will never yield to intellectual property rights, they simply are poor inventors and more easily lead as a head, whereas the Europanic has rugged individualism which leads to self sufficiency without the state involved. This is why we create Capitalist (and hopefully Libertarian) societies while asians has fallen to Monarchies (Japan until America stepped in, and Thailand until the Kings death) and Communism (China, North Korea, etc). The south Koreans show us that given the right push they can develop capitalist societies, invent, and prosper. But they don't get there themselves. It's the white mans burden, but the burden of saving the whole world has bankrupted America and led us down a frightening dysgenic path.

HISPANIC is not a race, it is a GOODY BAG of shakedowns for our government. disgusting. And it's on the American census as a racial category. This is horror. This is wrong. Italians and Germans have much stronger claims to being one people than Hispanics, yet THOSE are not recognized by the US government, even though both are much more rare minorities in America than Hispanics, and both groups have faced strong discrimination. For example, 20% of the US Population is Hispanic and 14% is black, but only 9% is Italian. So why don't Italians get minority status? Answer – BECAUSE THEY WORK FUCKING HARD.

So why do the Hispanics get all the goodies but we legislate racism AGAINST Italians and Germans? This is very wrong and evil. Our government in the USA is sick and run by the Gynocracy and oligarchs. These sick laws are created by the communists to destroy our nation and enable endless reckless breeding by the lesser races at the price of the HIGH IQ productive races. . It is disgusting.

Another mistake – They look at the genetic distance of Africans and Europanics and Asians and recognize this branch occurred a million years ago. But they say it was because we left Africa at that time. No, the out of Africa theory is utterly discredited in terms of races that developed in the 500,000 – 100,000 year ago time frame. We find these remains all over the world now. African americans seem to have more limited language and few words. Hence Rap Music – Fuck that NWORD cause I'm a whore NWORD, NWORD NWORD cap that ass NWORD" – No melody, no complex time swing out of the pocket, no modal harmonics, no 9ths, diminished chords, no 13ths. If we simply look at the music they create vs. Europanics it is so simply clear that this is a very diminished race. There are always a few outliers in any race – Blacks have Sowell, Nina Simone, Ellington, etc. But they are quite rare. And often of mixed blood as many American negros have 25-50% Europanic admixture. This is like super charging a car.

Lets look at the deep Africans to get a sense of the reality of the race without our European genes added to the mix and you get 70 IQs and hyper-violence. And this is what they are importing into Europe today. But if you recognize that most American blacks have a strong Eurpanic admixture often as much as 50% really they should be doing much much better than they are today. The racial pandering and affirmative action basically lets them keep not trying, the few who do try often end up Oprah rich.

In Guatemala, when the spanish left Antigua, all these beautiful churches which were damaged in an earthquake in the 1700s simply were left broken and rotten. The AmerInd race had no concept to understand complex architecture. Even the simple huts they live in on dirt floors are mostly built by NGO groups for them. With concrete and Aluminum sent from America. Because they have no understanding how to mine and create metals.

In Post Colonial Africa, many of these nations have lost the ability to run even the sewage and water systems built by the Europeans for them. Now they shit on the beaches. It all falls back to mud without the Europanics. Remember Lincoln pushed for the establishment of Liberia in Afrika and an exploratory group of Africans went over with Europanic Americans to help them build a civilization. Within a year the project had failed, Africans were starving and returning back to America. And the rest of the Africans stayed put in America, they know who butters their bread.

Zimbabwe starves and South Africa is next. The USA is broke because it is now saddled with 40% third world races. But **the births are already 51% negroid. Its a doom scenario. But recognizing that is called RACISM.**

So they flood the nation with Indians with fake degrees to replace our hard working engineers because they are "brown" so thats happy liberal snowflake prizes. Destroy the Europanic MALE! is the progressive war cry, and this is of course meant to put us on a path to doom and destruction from which the Commies hope to take over. That's WHY they are doing it, to destroy the great Europanic civilizations and evil ass-hats like Soros take their Jew won billions and push the destruction of Europanic nations.

WHY? Does he believe the MYTH of the HOLOHOAX and think that ergo proper hoc all white men are guilty? No he's far too smart for that. The reality is that the JEW has been the little man (physically shorter even) compared to the Europanic and if it weren't for the catholic church's smart ban on USURY they would have remained small. But they stepped in and corrupted the money systems and bankrupted kings and nations until they amassed all the wealth. Now our entire system is USURY based and DEBT SLAVE based. The jews won because the Europanic ruler could not stop his war lust, which is a trait hopefully we have somewhat bred out of us. But we survived because we were bloodthirsty killers and madmen. Sadly we have no survival instinct against money systems that enslave us.

We had nothing to do with India, no debts to that land. There is no reason for this except the Kalergi Plan and Communism – both Jewish constructions designed to enslave nations through racial deformity depravity and invasion. It is sick and it is violent. Millions die because of this horror. If you are afraid of being called a Racist when speaking the truth about these horrors then you are a weak pathetic cuck of a man not worthy of having a nation at all. We must stand up and reverse this NOW. If we don't want so many billions growing like weeds in Africa we must stop sending in hundreds of tons of free food for them every year. It is not draught, it is GENETIC DEPRAVITY and FAILURE of this race.

This assistance only grows more of them. And then they overflow and scream BOZZA (WELFARE!) as they seek a life of sitting on their ass and collecting free checks from the government. Are we really so stupid? Are we INSANE! This sickness of helping outside our race MUST END. It is a Jewish construct designed to bring in communism and enslave us. And to bankrupt us with endless welfare payments. WAKE UP. WAKE THE F-K UP.

The typical U.S. government form—where you're asked to fill in your ethnicity—differs depending on who issues it. But in general, the Liberal Elite's "Races of Man" are: White, Black, Hispanic (sometimes divided into Hispanic White and Hispanic Non-White), Asian, Pacific Islander and Native American. Sometimes, to make things even worse, you find options such as "Native American, Pacific Islander and Alaskan Native" or simply "API"—" Asian-Pacific Islander."

But in his soon-to-be-published book, *Race Differences in Psychopathic Personality,* British psychologist Professor Richard Lynn sets out a huge body of data implying that US race categories are simply not fit for purpose.

A "race", he tells us, is a breeding population separated long enough from another breeding population to have adapted to a different ecology, leading to consistent differences in average gene frequencies between the populations. This is important because, as Lynn shows, "race", therefore, expresses itself in consistent interrelated physical and mental differences, which tend to differ in the same direction because they are adaptations to distinct environments. Thus, different races have different genetic disease profiles, different dominant blood groups, different average IQ, and different modal personalities.

> I propose that the variable that explains these differences is that blacks are more psychopathic than whites. Just as racial groups differ in average IQ, they can also differ in average levels of other psychological traits, and racial differences in the tendency towards psychopathic personality would explain virtually all the differences in black and white behavior left unexplained by differences in IQ.
>
> Psychopathic personality is a personality disorder of which **the central feature is lack of a moral sense.** The condition was first identified in the early nineteenth century by the British physician John Pritchard, who proposed the term "moral imbecility" for those deficient in moral sense but of normal intelligence. The term psychopathic personality was first used in 1915 by the German psychiatrist Emile Kraepelin and has been employed as a diagnostic label throughout the twentieth century.
>
> In 1941 the condition was described by Hervey Cleckley in what has become a classic book, *THE MASK OF SANITY*. He **described the condition as general poverty of emotional feelings, lack of remorse or shame, superficial charm, pathological**

lying, egocentricity, a lack of insight, absence of nervousness, an inability to love, impulsive antisocial acts, failure to learn from experience, reckless behavior under the influence of alcohol, and **a lack of long-term goals.**

The Loss of the Europanic Peoples – No Homeland, Nowhere to Escape To, and the COST of the Spiteful Mutants will destroy us

When America falls it's game over. The last semi-free nation with our history of the Bill of Rights, a principal of freedom for its peoples, will have been extinguished.

Sadly, in times of prior crisis, Europeans fled to America. But there is no next hopping to nation to flee to. The fall of America will result in a global madness of petty wars and fights as trade lines dry up and smaller nations get gobbled by bullies.

It will be a return to a dark age. Perhaps we won't lose all knowledge like the fall or Rome, but we might.

The cost for the dysgenic transformation of the U.S.A from a Europanic nation with 9% non-europanics to a hodge podge society with 50% non-Europanics is shuttered upon the middle class in the form of property taxes.

Property taxes essentially turn America into a communist nation. There is no private property, everything is a loan from the state. That is exactly how they do it in China.

And rising property taxes are now required to support the huge pensions for the dumb people – the teachers, the police officers, the government workers, etc – while the smart hard working people generally are told "get a 401k" ha ha ha suckers.

The extreme welfare parasitism – ghetto mommas with ten chillin getting $2000 a month and a free house – and the refugee industry funnelling billions to the "charities" for housing and resettlement, and then the welfare comes. It's all adding to the massive taxes on the middle class. The Trump tax break? It didn't lower taxes. We lost the deduction for interest on mortgage and rates actually increased for the upper middle class, in exchange for a higher standard deduction. For most of the middle class it was a wash. the real benefits were of course given to the corporations.

But the low interest rates, which were caused from overspending on warfare and welfare which forces america to run at a 1 trillion dollar deficit each year – requires the low interest rates or America would be instantly bankrupt. But those same low interest rates make the 7% projected returns on the pension funds nearly impossible. Which is why the FED and FOMC pressured the largest corporations to use the corporate tax break to buy back stocks raising the markets and fluffing pension funds.

But at the municipal level, these pension costs leave them no recourse except to drive up property taxes. To a ridiculous level. And this is the doom of the middle class.

It's a complex dance. Many steps in between. So most people cannot understand that it is our move to a dysgenic welfare nation and prison nation of the poor genetics and high psychopathy races that all are a net drain on society, basically they overwhelm the Europanics production. 40% dysgenic was the tipping point and now we are at 50% dysgenic and running headlong into 70% dysgenic population by 2050. This is a doomsday scenario but much too complex for the regular American to follow.

Multi-culturalism, invasion, our welfare state, all must be changed. So what to do?

FIRST, end birthright citizenship recognition. It was never legally recognized and should not be the law. Trump can change this with a EO and a bureaucratic change.

SECOND, end ALL payola and welfare for invaders, illegals, and refugees UNTIL they obtain their green cards.

THIRD, change the welfare system so that there is a FIXED RATE regardless of the number of children AND a bonus to women for not having any children.

That is not enough to save us, but it will slow down the ghetto-ization of America. And maybe as we watch Sweden fail and burn to the ground we might just wake up and restore our Europanic nation.

An even more equitable solution would be to end welfare altogether, and every American who earns under $200k would have the option to request $1000 a month. Many wouldn't take the money. But, and this is where the Yang Gang FAILS, is that you must then end all welfare, section 8, food stamps, money for "chillin" AND on top of that you have to stop giving disability for having an IQ which is representative of your race. We cannot give out disability payola if you are negro and have a 80 IQ because that is normal. Also, disability payola must be based on a working income for the average of the past 10 years. If you haven't put in 10 years, no disability. That would stop asians importing their grandmothers and mothers and immediately putting them on disability roles.

And of course, if you aren't a citizen you get NADA. Green card holder? NADA. And of course that leads us to BirthRight citizenship reform, which NEVER existed as a law and NO the 14th amendment doesn't confer it. You must have ONE PARENT who is an American Citizen to confer citizenship on the child.

All of this has to happen all together. And much of it can be done via executive order as much of this is administrative and reflects the payola back to the states for welfare. If a state like CAli wants to bankrupt itself by handing out welfare payments to illegal invaders, so be it, but no more Obama bailouts to California like we have done in the past.

The Democrats switched from standing up for social assistance programs and the working class / union to embracing Jacobsonian Progressivism which is basically Bolshevik Communism designed to break nations and take them over.

Already more than 50% of our births are to non-Europanics so already without a direction change it's only a matter of time before America collapses. We have sadly, already lost.

But that doesn't mean they will stop flooding America with brown dysgenic races. What the central American's do not understand that while they think they are flee-ing violence and gangs, it is their very GENETICS that create that kind of a nation. So they will forever bring that horror with them no matter where they go. Not every person. But it's imprinted in their DNA to be less able to form trusting stable societies. The same is true of Africanized genetics whether Somali, Congolese, or Middle Eastern. They can only express a level of civilization because then several factors begin to take over – levels of rape violence, inability to respect or think morally. We consider things like the Burkha and the violent repressive iron fist governments that run these places, and their iron fisted controlling religion – to be horrific to the freedom western minded. But That is precisely what is REQUIRED to control a population of non-Europanics. They are simply lower on the societal evolutionary scale. If you find that distressing, please cite a nation that is representative which is a net producer, provides a social safety net, and health care.

When you bring in millions upon millions of that element you get what we see in the streets of America today – violence, rapes, lack of social cohesion, people on welfare, and people in jail – as the dying Europanic society desperately tries to maintain a standard that the people no longer are capable of. It's like how in Liberia they lost the knowledge of how to repair and run the sewage systems, and then all the people just started shitting on the beaches – forever ruining the one source of high economy they might have had – tourism.

The Democratic plan is to shit on our beach. How they mean to do it is rather obvious.

1. Push for invasion invasion invasion by non-Europanics. It's called the Kalergi plan.
2. Recognize invaders as the same as citizens in as many ways as possible
3. Count the invaders in the census to claim congressional seats (see California)
4. Push for Drivers licenses for illegal (that finally fell in California) in 2013 under Traitor Brown and Comrade Kamala
5. Have voter registration forms with the drivers license forms. Most illegals won't have a clue they aren't legal to vote, and they will fill them out and not vote.
6. Pass "ballot dumping" laws so that you can literally go to a poll station and dump a truckload of ballots all for people not associated with you in any way
7. Run a cross check of illegal voter registrations vs. legal. Print out absentee ballots for all the illegals and mark them democrat.
8. When polls close, kick out all non democratic operative, review the voter polls for non-votes, and fill in ballots for them all voting DEMOCRATIC. This happens in every major city in a swing state like Arizona, Iowa.
9. Oppose all voter ID laws and bring busses that go to every voting place one after another and vote over and over under different names (in states without ballot dumping)
10. When the president ORDERS a review of Ballots, SIMPLY REFUSE to hand them over

Sound's horrific? IT"S BEEN HAPPENING FOR 20 YEARS NOW!

While the Democrats endlessly cheat, the Republicans more or less play a general trickster game, but not with the whole handed cheating and fake votes and plying the illegal aliens as voter pawns that the Democrats have engineered.

The numbers are frightening. In 2019 we are releasing into America more than 40,000 Illegal aliens every month due to overcrowding – the Emergency on the Border. It is estimated that it is 1.5 MILLION a year. Add the 1.5 Million in legal immigrants (including the 350,000 Software scab labor who pour in with fake degrees on the genocidal H-1B visa that no one ever cares about) and we have total death of a nation.

Well what's the problem what's the big deal, we will just become a majority negro (by that I mean non-europanic) nation. Except, we do not find productivity and work ethic in these peoples. The black model is atrocious, ending up in welfare, prison, or an aborted pile of goo at Planned Parenthood. The Hispanic model is slightly more devious with the 15 year old wife marrying a 40 year old man and having 3 babies by the time they are 19. Then the wife goes on welfare, we treat the babies as American citizens, and in places like california they get free breakfast, lunch, dinner, housing, education, they get to file for 18,000 in back earned income credit, and they get free healthcare. All of that is if they work through what is LEGAL and that's a big IF. Meanwhile, the "husband" who is not listed as the husband, lives in the section 8 housing, makes more babies, and works mostly in cash only jobs like lawns, construction, painting, and even if they do have to produce W-4 signed sworn statements of identity they just lie because they are NEVER PROSECUTED FOR IT! NEVER!

One set of rules for the invaders, and a different harsher set for the Europanic citizens. Being on welfare is the winning path to have babies because the Europanic workers are so exhausted and overtaxed the thought of being ready for babies and a household seems impossible. So they put it off. And Maybe by forty they have one baby. Meanwhile the black woman has 15 babies from 15 daddies and the Hispanic woman is nearly as bad and all of them find plenty of time to lounge around, watch TV and make more babies.

Financially we are already at 1.5 TRILLION a year overspending to keep this massive social system afloat and the projections look terrible. Doctors, refusing to BUDGE ONE INCH on their salaries routinely earn over $400,000 a year with many professions like cardiology and neuro surgery earning well in front of $800,000 a year. This "MEDICAL EXTORTION TAX" finds its way into EVERY ASPECT OF COSTS IN AMERICA including prices of all our products, property taxes, everything. The whole system is horribly uncompetitive because of this and China makes products for 10 cents on our dollar. Which is why we cannot make anything in America anymore. Which is why Yeezy sneakers (I know little about this ghetto affectation) cost $400 a pair.

Financially the costs to provide all these welfare programs are overwhelming the system and worse remove benefits for the hard working Europanic population. We are seeing this in all nations that are being invaded – cutbacks in Sweden and Germany and France about as well. And the forever money printing to cover our fall shorts each year, produce a 10% a year inflation that they call somehow 2.3 %. (see ShadowStats for a bit closer to the truth numbers). Do you feel poorer each year? This is why. And it's all because the nation is becoming non-productive non-europanic or, more simply said, precisely like the nations the invaders came from.

The problem is, America ALREADY had a massive dysgenic burden to handle from its huge numbers of black people who were slave descendents (although nowadays that's probably less than 50% of them). They have grown from 9% to 14%. Wait if they are poor how is that possible? If they get tons of abortions how is that possible? It's the welfare racket and on the other side, outrageous affirmative action and race hustling and everything free for blacks – college, sports cars, million dollar basketball salaries. Blacks are doing great! As long as the Europanics keep slaving 80 hour weeks to pay for them.

At some point, the host nation recognizes the PARASITE and says enough. If you are riddled with worms, a some point you put a gun to your head and say I don't care I can't go on. White men have been ridden like cows and milked until they are bone dry. Shrivled up mummies now they be. And as there is no way to fight the system, the only answer you could possibly give, is to take your beautiful Europanic brain and skills and go somewhere else.

And then, THEN you will find barrier after barrier. Want to move to mexico and get permanent residency? You will have to prove an income of $2500 a month or show $100,000 in investments of they will put you in JAIL. Wait, why doesn't America have the same thing. Why don't we have interior enforcement, why don't we charge illegals with perjury for lying on their W-4s, faking federal IDs, all of that would put a Europanic in jail for more than TEN YEARS. Nope, they get away with it. Two tiered justice system. Actually three, the illegals get off scott free, Europanic Americans get sent to jail over the tiniest of infraction, and the Hillary Clintons of the world also get off scott free. And at that point it's not my country any more. I just want out. I bet you do too. We have taken the political approach to the end electing Trump and he has done NOTHING. He could easily:

1) Declare that in order to get a social security number we require a SSN from one of your parents. That's an executive order. Take it to the supreme court

2) Declare that on matters of national security it requires a SUPREME COURT to overrule him. Thats the correct interpretation of equal powers.

3) Begin jailing illegal aliens for being here and overstaying visas. Then throwing them out.

4) Hire 5,000 amnesty "judges" no not full lawyers, just people who they give a 2 week training course to, and then we could be processing 250,000 cases a WEEK not a decade. There is NO LAW that says amnesty requests need to be vetted by LAWYERS.

Well you get the gist of it. Siezing voting records from California and finally proving they had millions of fake illegal voters, arresting and jailing Hillary Clinton, Comey, Rosenstein, Obama, and all the other traitors would help. A full hard court offensive is required to turn the death ship around. But it AINT HAPPENING! So… sorry my nation of my birth, I am not wanton to be part of the blood bath to come, I am leaving you.

A healthy Europanic society can ONLY SUPPORT 10% Negroid populations. Any more than that and we go broke.

White Per Capita$2,795

Black Per Capita-$10,016

Hispanic Per Capita-$7,298

These numbers do not include PRISON costs.

At the end of 2016, federal and state prisons in the United States held about 486,900 inmates who were black and 439,800 who were white – a difference of 47,100, according to BJS.There were 339,300 hispanics in prison in that year.

In 2016, blacks represented 12% of the U.S. adult population but 33% of the sentenced prison population. Whites accounted for 64% of adults but 30% of prisoners. And while Hispanics represented 16% of the adult population, they accounted for 23% of inmates.

Think we can re-elect Trump ? Think again.

the total cost per inmate averaged $33,274 in 2015 (https://www.vera.org/publications/price-of-prisons-2015-state-spending-trends/price-of-prisons-2015-state-spending-trends/price-of-prisons-2015-state-spending-trends-prison-spending)

White Prison Cost: 14.6 Billion

Black Prison Cost: 16.2 Billion

Hispanic Prison Cost: 11.3 Billion

So Impact of Whites is 539.9 Billion

Blacks: – 405.92 Billion

Hispanics: – 423.3 Billion

Black + Hispanic Cost to the Nation Each Year: 829.21 BILLION

It shows already at 62% White the cost of having spiteful mutants subsume us has placed us 289 BILLION in debt every year. corporate taxes only add 225 BILLION. Leaving 64 BILLION in deficit.

Our discretionary spending part of the budget is 1,200,000,000,000 dollars. The cost of dysgenics leave 64,000,000,000 dollars to pay for all that. Is it any wonder we are running a trillion+ dollar deficit EACH YEAR?

What does that do? It causes INFLATION – 10% a year inflation, which WRECKS the white middle class and makes saving your way out of poverty IMPOSSIBLE. Then they offer NO INTEREST ON DEPOSITS. It's a double f-k. All because of our spiteful mutants.

Getting Europanic Women to have Babies in a Broken World

If we formed a break away society, a new mini-state, we would need a new plan, a new way of doing things. Here are some ideas.

One of the biggest issues we have fallen into is this notion of delayed childhood for women. Women in Mexico have their Quencerana (15 year old coming out party) after which they are "fair game" for partnering up and marriage. Age of consent was 14 to 16 in many states, but they have all been changed to … apparently 30 years of age to "protect the children". Indeed women are seen as children, yet with full equality, well past the years of child rearing. This needs to change.

Instead we should return to the traditional coming out party at 15, but with a difference. A cast of suitors would apply to each woman and a council of elders would have to approve them. They would have to have established themselves as hard workers and productive. No slackers going on college loans getting the good women. From this pool of say 100 at the part, the men would give the women their cards with their bios, introduce themselves, chat and dance. The woman then has to make a selection of five. Each of these five would then accept the woman for a one month trial marriage. There would be no sex no touching, simply see if they could co-habitate. This would continue and if the woman reached the end of her five to no avail, could then pick her second set of five. But by then she must choose. Her primary duty to society is to marry and raise children. At least four, preferably SIX. Because the new society is directly in competition against the larger crass broken systems population growth is a must. Women who reach eight or more children are honored with a special gold star they get to pin on their vests and all other women must respect them as honored.

Men on the other hand would work until 30. establish themselves. And not date. They would understand that comes later. After taking on a first wife, every ten years they would be allowed to take on another if they can prove they have the finances for it. Productive men will get a steady stream of beautiful women to marry at 16 and have them until 26 when they will switch (the women that is) over to raising the children and preparing the household. So a very productive man might have 3 wives and 18 children. The wives however, also get something special. After having at least 4 children and raising them to the age of 16 (their age being 35 or 36) they have the option to leave the household giving the husband one year to find a new wife of 16. Then if they want to be career women they can begin their education and pursue life however they wish. They will wear the bronze star as recognition that they are free of their wifely obligations and have completed their family raising. They will also receive a one time small sum from the household they leave to begin their new life, say $20,000. Which they would have planned for with a saving account depositing $1000 into it every year.

This really does allow everyone the best of both worlds. Men get to pursue their careers and be productive, have children, and wife or wives to take care of the home front. Women still get to pursue careers once they are done.

And what of the leftover people who are not qualified to marry or work productive jobs. Well they will get the menial jobs and the men will also have the option to go on to the military and establish themselves that way.

Another thing which needs a big rethink is paying taxes. Taxes should be paid when you are dead. 50% of the household would go to the children, and the other 50 to taxes. There should be no taxation holding you back in life. Wealth would have to be registered and could not be blown away on lavish lifestyles the few years before death. Which brings us to…

Medical. One of the reasons why doctors are SOOO ridiculously expensive in America is because we force them to go to school twice. Again treating people like children. This is not the norm around the world. At 16 they should be able to go on and study medine and by 20 qualify to practice. Then they can part time do a specialty internship for an advanced dicipline while still seeing patients. Poor but smart kids could get scholarship to be doctors providing they work 10 years in the free clinics before going onto private practice. And the free clinics would be where many would get a basic checkup, prescription, or broken bone mended.

Guns. Everyone would be trained in the use of guns and all men of 25 years or older would be require to holster a gun on their hip at all times. Anti society crimes like robbery, theft, violence could all be responded to by anyone with a gun. The need for police and prisons would be smaller. And people shot committing a crime would not get free medical care if any.

Drugs. All drugs would be legal. But addicts would be eventually forced into either Ibogaine (or the lesser large dose psilocybin) recovery centers. This treatment ends the addictive cravings. But America being so stupid and anti-drug cannot consider it.

Homeless/End of Life Care: If despite all our efforts you have ended up homeless then you would be wafted over to our Enjoyment centers where fed an ever increasing dose of the purest morphines you would relax away the final weeks of life with gourmet food, music, and entertainment. Then you'd become dog food. A similar treatment would be given for the feeble but as long as they were self financially viable they could opt out and continue aging as long as they wish.

Property Taxes: All property taxes would be illegal. Education would be charged for or people could home school and formal home schooling programs and software would be designed and free from the state.

Education: Education would be all self paced. With most people expected to complete to 10th year level by age 16 in order to enter normal society. College education would only exist for medicine, law, and the hard sciences, with all other degrees being done online.

Immigration: All new people who seek to come into the society would have to pass a group of elders screening and these would be elected by each community of 1000 – 10 elders. Applicants would be screened and have to pass the 10th grade tests before being allowed in. One issue is would non-Europanics be allowed in this society and yes, they could be, with controlled numbers not to exceed 10% and only those showing great merits – amazing scientists, doctors, musicians, and cooks. All these merits would be specifically tested and qualified by similar councils of elders for each merit area.

Government. Five people of good standing would be chosen entirely by random for each council of elders group. They would all be vetted to minimum requirements by the elders. Then the public at large would vote. The male of each household would represent the vote for that household. It's not that women aren't allowed to vote, but they should make their voice part of that households vote. The bronze star women who have left a successful household and are now in careers can also vote independently. The number of female voters would always be kept at a subset of the male, keeping a soft patriarchy firmly entrenched. This would happen naturally as most women aged 16-36 will be under the male household and only some would leave. As we have learned from the USA and Europe, Gynocracy left to it's own accord eventually spins out of control and exterminates societies. So that cannot be allowed to happen again. So say the population of the new state is 10 million. That's 10,000 individual councils who each would field one candidate. Then ten states, each of a million person size, would begin the process of debates and run off of the candidates until the final ten were obtained who would then be given totally free air time each week to speak to the people so that raising money was no longer needed. These would be chosen at random into pairs of 2 for one on one debates lasting one hour each until each person had debated several other candidates. The group debates of 17 people simply is useless. One on one debating requires thinking and mental sparing and really showing the merits of your ideas.

With the president chosen, the remaining next 10 scoring candidates would be added to the council for a 10 year appointment, and the 10 oldest members of the congressional will retire out. There would be no parties, no groups fighting against each other, just a society of individuals, chosen by the people. A republic just as the USA is, a constitutional republic bound by laws. We can keep the first 10 amendments more or less, the rest are pretty much trash.

financially, as a society within a society all of this would be made clear to those who joined but protecting our members from the external taxation and militaries of the outer society would be nearly impossible. A piece of land would have to be taken militarily, preferably an island, and with nuclear technology being quite simple to understand by intellectual types, building our nuclear arsenal would be an immediate step before things became too public. Following the Israeli model we would claim religious need for our own state and anyone who speaks out against us as religious persecution. Call them Anti-White-ites. err something like that.

Currency: Fiat currency would be abandoned for gold-notes, which could always be exchanged (up to some fairly large limit to prevent fat cats from absconding with gold) into gold at any bank. Banks would make their money from traditional loaning and interest rates would probably be a bit higher to give them enough profits, but it would never be a multiplier of gold reserves it would be 1:1. So while an american bank has $1M in deposit and can make $50M in loans, our banks would only be able to make $800,000 in loans with the rest being working capital reserves. Corporate stocks, stock markets, and raising capital would all work how they do now.

Trade: There would be a moral system of tariff for all goods coming in starting at 10% base tariff. this would fund the government. Extra tariff penalties for nations that don't respect property rights or labor conditions until finally countries like China would fail so many of they tests they wouldn't be allowed as trading partners at all

Energy: Advanced safer nuclear designs like salt thorium reactors would be the main game in town, along with solar for electric and cracking water into hydrogen using high frequencies to drive cars. Cars would be hydrogen or electric with removable batteries, and batteries would be exchanged at a system of fuel stations. No plugs. No gasoline. The USA has blocked advanced nuclear design research for decades instead preferring their bomb based water cooled high pressure designs like Fukushima reactors. Madness.

I like to think of the USA as a first experiment, this would be the second. Having learned the lessons from many countries attempts at democracy, this would surely be an improvement.

How to Face the Collapse of the USA ?

One of the things that happens when confronted with the thought that your nation is on a runaway freight train collision course to obliteration, is to realize that this has been going on for several decades. At some point you have to shrug off the seriousness of the battle and build productive lives. One of the important things is to keep your sense of humor and laughter.

Nietzsche has a few things to say on laughter. Nietzsche's time was a similar time when mankind was repressed, for him, by a false Christian morality, the herd morality. It was a control mechanism that the powerful wrought and used to turn men into slaves.

This is most powerfully illustrated by Zarathustra's vision near the start of part three in *Thus Spake Zarathustra*. Within this vision, following the first explicit presentation of eternal recurrence, to his great enemy the 'Spirit of Gravity', Zarathustra is confronted with a young shepherd into whose mouth a heavy black snake has entered and bitten into the shepherd's throat.

Try as he might, Zarathustra cannot tug the snake from the agonized shepherd, so he urges him to bite off its head. The shepherd .. . bit as my cry had advised him; he bit with a good bite! He spat far away the snake's head — and sprang up. No longer a shepherd, no longer a man—a transformed being, surrounded with light, laughing.

Never yet on earth had any man laughed as he laughed! 0 my brothers, I **heard a laughter that was no human laughter—and now a thirst consumes me, a longing that is never stilled. My longing for this laughter consumes me: oh how do I endure still to live! And how could I endure to die now!**

Zarathustra cannot endure to die now because he has not yet laughed this extraordinary laughter. The urge to do so drives

him on, and eventually, his consuming thirst is quenched, the real culmination of the book coming in the final four sections of the third part. Indeed, Zarathustra's facing up to and finally embracing his most 'abysmal thought' – the eternal recurrence.

In a mindset of DOOM the eternal recurrence is a horrific death sentence. That this terrible path will repeat over and over.

But in mindset of YEA-saying to the universe, the eternal recurrence is an AFFIRMATION of standing against the universe and YELLING YOUR WILL against it. I AM ALIVE AND THIS IS MY WILL!

You can think of Schopenhauer " Die Welt als Wille und Vorstellung" The world as will and idea. Embracing that the universe is a product of your will, and your ideas engender its existence, make manifest your spirit.

The rules exist to herd the lower man. They are told THOU SHALT and humble and kneel blindly following their masters and the roles that this current society permutation has given them. Heidegger called it THROWN-ness. You are cast into the Universe beset with the rules of the current permutation.

Are you willing to sell your ghost for the sake of some uniform standard?

But the rules are made to be bent and broken, crushed through by the exalted men. The rare person of will and strength who stands against the winds of the Universe and says I SHALT. And the greatest of men not only push society forward with their accomplishments but literally PUSH THE RULE FRAMEWORK of society forward as well. This is the ultimate trick of living. And this is what ultimately dispels the doom cycle. So while we stare at our eventual societal collapse, the new re-envisioning by these strong spirited people will take root. Seedlings. But quickly grow and devour with a new standard.

One can think of the early Christians against the Roman empire. The empire all powerful, kept killing them. They were heretics.

But eventually the emperor Constantine asked, hmmm, what is it with these Christians that they seem to have such power of spirit? And then Christianity was embraced.

Right now we are a society reeling from a destructive list of concepts that seem to build upon each other – Universal College, No free land, Welfare, Feminism, Endless Immigration and racial replacement. We have become a non-society, simply an agglomeration of people stuck in a place with no other free-er land to leave to. Somehow we have to begin the difficult process of being free somehow somewhere someway. What that is no one can claim to know, but it will begin. It is the RESPONSE to the horror that has been pushed upon us by masters that have been too greedy.

Think of the USA in the 1750s. People fed up with Tyranny against the strongest army ever know – the British. Should they have had any hope whatsoever of success? Samuel Adams and Thomas Paine and even Benjamin Franklin, The Sons of Liberty movement, all grew until eventually the landed gentry had to consider it all and make a decision. With everything to lose, they chose to shrug off tyranny. That's almost unthinkable today. But only when there are enough great men to act can society change. Unfortunately even the freedom that was fought for is now nearly stolen and our societies light of liberty extinguished. The elections are frauds, and our economics are those of enslavement. Who will do something? They have machine guns and atomic bombs, does human existence end in total slavery?

The Rise of the Spiteful Mutants is important to recognize, because unless we work against that we will get engulfed by them and conquered. Like Neo in the Matrix covered in goo. We lose the ability to speak or protest. We are swallowed whole.

At the end of part three, we discover that the young shepherd with the snake is Zarathustra himself.

" The great disgust at man-il choked me and had crept into my throat: and what the prophet prophesied: 'It is all one, nothing is worth while, knowledge chokes'.... 'Alas, man recurs eternally! The little man recurs eternally!' had seen them both naked, the greatest man and the smallest man: all too similar to one another, even the greatest all too human! The greatest all too small!—that was my disgust at man! And eternal recurrence even for the smallest! that was my disgust at all existence!16 Eternal recurrence is such an 'abysmal thought' because, if everything eternally recurs, this includes that which is small in man, which Nietzsche so passionately loathes. 'Nothing is worth while' because the ideal of a future Obermensch, it seems, cannot be realized.

Confronted with this thought, Zarathustra is so sickened that he is unable to get up, eat or drink for seven days. **So how is this sickness triumphed over: how may the snake's head be bitten off? The answer, as Zarathustra comes to realize, is to give the highest affirmation of life possible: to say a joyous Yes to life despite its negative side, despite its horrors and suffering.**

"And we should consider every day lost on which we have not danced at least once. And we should call every truth false which was not accompanied by at least one laugh."

How do we fight these non-truths that society has adopted? "Not by wrath does one kill, but by laughter." Ultimately when we all laugh at them in their faces at the PREPOSTERITY of their ideas, on that day our shackles break and we are freed. This is why the LEFT is so anti-humor and decries it all "hate speech" REE REE "hate speech!" like some besotted parrot. When their tangled mess of ideas becomes so obviously ridiculous we will laugh and laugh each time they speak until they become red-faced. This is why the controlled news is so dangerous, they spew and spew without an audience, an immunity from the laughter and derision we would – as sane men and women – heap upon them.

We live in a time where the pill has engendered a new enslavement of man in marriage such that we simply laugh at it. Ridiculous. It's like Harry Potter. RIDICULOUS and the phantom cannot survive.

The tricky part is this morass is all consuming all around us. New frontiers and bastions and bulwarks have yet to be built. "I'd like to buy some free land please" and they laugh at US – RIDICULOUS. This just accepting it has to change. Buy a RV not a house. If we no longer can have free land then no land we shall have. Run off to an island. Stop playing by THEIR rules. Better rules and better rule-sets will take over, but not in our lifetime. It's going to be a lot of general collapse and suffering. Like the fall of Czarist Russia. We can"t stop living our life by our rules and our beliefs and wait for change. We simply must object and seek alternatives as much as they present themselves.

If the educational system is so bereft of real education, then again, RIDICULOUS. There's no point in continuing to attend simply for that Harvard Stamp on our foreheads affirming we have somehow passed some now communist standard. RIDICULOUS.

If the women are not loving and giving and seeking children in their child years and instead want to come back at 35 after riding the male carousel for 20 years, RIDICULOUS.

If they want to import 100 million immigrants and throw the natives away, and then deliver us TAX bills on everything to pay for these unproductive Spiteful Mutants – RIDICULOUS.

If they want to import 4 million Indians and Chinese with fake degrees to take the software engineer jobs – 100% replacement of our best and brightest. RIDICULOUS. It is designed to make us feel defeated. It is designed to break our wills. It is designed for the unproductive MBAs to cackle and feel superior as they throw their productive people away. Eventually it will have consequences.

If they re-write all our heroes as pregnant lesbian woke avengers RIDICULOUS. Don't watch the movies or buy the comics. This is created to entertain the Spiteful Mutants, not us.

Like the movie Wargames, at some point the best move to play is not the play the game at all. At some point, pressure will build. There have to be alternatives. We can find them. Sadly the tax system America has declared, is now upon you no matter WHERE you live in the world. If that alone doesn't tell you we are living under slavery nothing will.

In the end we are all too human. But that humanity is also our salvation. We are the inventors and we are the mindful creators. We have a joyous spirit and can laugh at the universe. And each day, undefeated, we can YEA-say one word. ONWARD!

When I was a teen and young adult, life confused me. I thought I must be insane. And the girls and fiancees that I met all convinced me that there must be something terribly wrong with me. But when I grew older, I came to realize that nearly everyone else was insane, and I was the sane one in a world gone mad. It's a sinking feeling. Not one of joy nor accomplishment. But, once you realize that, you are unstoppable. The others lose their power. And you realize yourself. And the spiteful mutants? They change. No longer monsters and terrors destroying your world, they become pitiable tragic creatures. And you walk away from worrying.]

We are in the throws of the Yugi-kalpa, the dark times. But it's ever so odd that everyone pretends not to see it. Everything that is happening is a symptom of this crescendo growing louder and yet dumber and dumber people keep talking on the television telling us this is life as normal. It is a cycle that must be completed there is no sense to try and stop it. The snake does not bother you any more. You realize it is ok that the overman is not reached, OK that the lowerman is still bound, OK in the face of recurrence. You are empowered in a world that is blind. Finally free, you chart your own path. A slow laughter pervades your soul.

Conclusion: Two Futures Await Us

The first future is the return to a soft patriarchy. Men work in the world and women keep the home and produce many babies and only consider returning to work after raising them all to 14 is completed. Perhaps a small percentage of exceptional women are given passes to pursue careers straight off after passing exams and live unmarried as an analogue to the MGTOW men, but not many. Cars are brilliant and amazing, houses gleam and are affordable, and the new six hour day four day workweek lets people rest enough to always give the next week its all. Rather than the old 50 – 52 work weeks a year, America has reformed itself such that there are 4 weeks of flexible vacation plus one month in summer. Doctors go straight to medical school and skip college so medical costs are lower. Freedoms increase and our pioneer spirit slowly returns as the dysgenic fractured races either LEAVE or reform themselves due to the lack of welfare. Welfare, true welfare would require first TEN YEARS of work, and then be based on your total tax contribution during that time. No more high school girls getting pregnant to get free housing and dollars. Crime goes way down and cities re-bloom. A new pioneer spirit and can do and inventions appear that are amazing. We are no longer isolated and alone, but instead walk in a brotherhood of men.

The second future the fat hippo feminists win. All movies are de-masculinized and women with few skills take on roles like doctor and engineer leading to many deaths and bridge collapses. The nation embraces socialism and debt, and welcomes immigrants from the whole world to come live here, driving taxes through the roof and housing prices. Water is scare and fresh food is unheard of. People end up living in tiny horror boxes and the streets are dangerous after ICE was disbanded and the police were replaced by the new "Help force". FAT is the new sexy and the reproduction rate plummets to near ZERO. Only the dysgenics on welfare breed producing a dumb society that can no longer fix the modern "JEDI" services they cannot understand. Sewage runs in the street. Eventually the Chinese and the Mongols arrive to take over. The Hispanics sell them burritos. Women who are thin or young are rounded up and put into sex slave barges back to the yellow homelands while the fat hippo women are shot for pig food. The native men are shot but a few flee south to establish new societies that never allow spiteful mutants and feminists to take over ever again. The nation ceases to exist and the new Chinese/Mongol hordes establish a strict patriarchy where women live only in chains. Well ladies, you asked for it.

Printed by BoD™in Norderstedt, Germany